Fructose Malabsorption
The Survival Guide

Debra & Bob Ledford

Debra's Dedication

To my husband and co-author, Bob, without whose love and support this book and my current state of wellness would not have been possible.

Bob's Dedication

To my wife, Debra, for her willingness to open her mind and her eagerness to share what she has learned to help others.

Table of Contents

Introduction

When I was first diagnosed in January 2007 with Fructose Malabsorption (FM), the extreme frustration we felt trying to find sources of information was exasperating. Numerous hours on the internet produced insignificant help, only confusing us more. The few lists available were conflicting, without explanations. We saw the need for a single, reliable source.

After perhaps thousands of hours of research, we compiled what we felt at the time was the most comprehensive resource available for the FM sufferer. Thankfully, much has been learned over the last twelve years, with less conflicting information now available. In this updated Second Edition we have attempted to address: questions asked by the FMer, current lists, resources, living with FM from an FMer's point of view, dealing with the effects, recipes, our viewpoints, and much more.

If you have comments, questions, corrections, recommendations, or other helpful information, please e-mail us at dledford11@gmail.com. We may include it in future editions of this book.

Disclaimer

This is a book written by an FM couple as support for FMers and their families. We are not medical professionals and are not qualified to dispense advice, medical or otherwise. The information contained herein is a compilation of research and our opinions, not meant to be taken as medical advice. We urge you to consult your physician and get tested before implementation of anything contained in this book.

My Story – Part One

As a preface to my story, I would like to advise my readers that out of necessity of subject matter, I will be sharing very personal information. I do this, not from lack of sensitivity or discretion, but to better facilitate understanding of this condition and its effect on me.

Approximately thirteen years ago, I began my journey of discovery into the cause behind the stomach problems I was experiencing. What had previously been chronically irritating problems had become an acutely disruptive condition. Stomach pain was almost constant, I purchased antacids in large quantities, uncontrollable flatulence provided a source of humiliation, and severe constipation made me ill.

With constipation seeming to be the primary source of my misery, I focused on it. Aware that regular laxative use can create a physical dependence, I began with more natural and pleasant methods. I love fruit, so I focused on oranges, the only fruit which had ever aided me with constipation. Adding prune juice, despite it never providing me the same results digestively which it apparently does the general population, helped to appease those attempting to advise me. I also focused on high-fiber foods, grains, and vegetables, which are purported to aid digestion. I also increased my water intake, although I tend to drink large amounts anyway. Additionally, I avoided meats, cheese, milk, and other products which might be slowing my processing facilities. Despite all of this, matters just got worse.

3

As a lifelong opponent of fad diets, desperate describes what I was feeling and my next course of action. I resorted to a liquid-only diet in an attempt to go. In addition to broth and plenty of water, this meant fruit and vegetable juices. As a health-conscious parent, I had always required all juice consumed in our home to be 100% juice, without added sweeteners or flavors, so be assured, this juice was actually juice. All to no avail, the earth still moved, but I did not.

For those who have never known the experience of chronic and severe constipation, after about three weeks, the toxins accumulate within the body to the extent one becomes quite ill, take-to-your-bed type ill. I was nearing this. Extreme situations–as they say–so I bought what I felt would be the strongest over-the-counter laxative I could get, Extra-Strength Ex-Lax. I took the maximum dosage for a full week. Not only was I surprised I did not experience the usual cramping such products cause, but this also resulted in an insignificant amount of action.

After making an appointment with an internist and having blood tests, his nurse telephoned, stating the tests were all normal, and the doctor had called in a prescription for a laxative. I would not need to return. I said, "No, thank you." I was not interested in only treating the symptoms; I wanted to know the cause. I demanded a referral to a gastroenterologist, a specialist of the digestive tract. A few days later I went for my appointment.

At the gastroenterologist's, the nurse practitioner took an extensive medical history, as well as details of my current problem. More tests were ordered to discover if the acid reflux had caused esophageal damage and to rule out such things as Crohn's disease and colitis, both hereditary diseases which my brother was diagnosed with at the age of twenty-one. However, she felt there was a good possibility I might have fructose malabsorption. After being told it is an intolerance to fructose, I was determined this was not my problem. After all, I love fruits and vegetables.

After a wonderfully liberating week of a combination of different laxatives, I went back for more tests, one of which tested for fructose malabsorption. The good news that all the tests showed me to be perfectly healthy was overshadowed by the fact that the nurse practitioner had been correct; I have fructose malabsorption.

What is Fructose Malabsorption?

With fructose malabsorption (FM), erroneously known as fructose intolerance or dietary fructose intolerance, fructose, a naturally occurring sugar found in fruit, vegetables, and honey, is not absorbed by the small intestine. Normally, fructose is absorbed by the small intestine using enterocytes—intestinal absorptive cells—to break up molecules and transport them into the tissues. In those for whom this protein is missing, inactive, or reduced, the fructose continues to the large intestine, where it is fermented by intestinal bacteria becoming short-chain fatty acids and the gases carbon dioxide, methane, and hydrogen.

If you're wondering why you have never heard of FM, you're not alone. It is a somewhat recent diagnosis. This does not mean it is the latest fad diagnosis. This means until recently, it was unknown what caused this group of symptoms.

Important: *fructose malabsorption should not be confused with hereditary fructose intolerance* (HFI), a rare, life-threatening disorder in which fructose is absorbed within the small intestine but is not metabolized by the liver. HFI is a completely different condition unrelated to FM. People with this disorder require a completely fructose-free diet.

Causes of Fructose Malabsorption

Unfortunately, the exact cause of FM is unknown. Most researchers theorize it is caused by the excessive amounts of fructose which we consume in today's society. One trip through the grocery store to read labels will leave a person asking why everything we eat must have some form of sugar, especially high fructose corn syrup (HFCS).

Another theory is the overuse of antibiotics. Unfortunately, antibiotics are non-discriminatory. Though they can do a great job of killing the harmful bacteria which make us sick, they are also busy attacking and destroying good bacteria. The body is a delicate balance of bacteria, yeast, and other beastly things. By reducing the good bacteria in our bodies through the use of antibiotics, we throw that balance off. This is why a bacterial infection is often followed by a yeast infection. What is to keep these potent drugs (antibiotics), which we may also be getting from their overuse in our meats and dairy, from destroying other essential body elements such as enzymes and enterocytes?

Some wonder if FM could be hereditary. While we must reiterate that FM must not be confused with Hereditary Fructose Intolerance (HFI), this does not mean FM could not also be hereditary. A little time spent on any support group site can reveal this possibility. If it were not hereditary or at least predisposed in families, why do we see families with several members who have FM?

Just as genetic makeup predisposes some people to obesity, alcoholism, and diabetes, perhaps our genetics may increase the likelihood of FM in our families. To follow this a bit further, just as with obesity, alcoholism, or diabetes, perhaps a careful diet for those predisposed to FM may help to prevent it.

Yet another theory is the extensive use of pesticides, herbicides, and other alterations to our foods. If these processes are meant to kill organisms, what is to keep them from killing the organisms and delicate body parts we all need to function normally? Almost every food we eat has been sprayed with something, or several things, and/or altered in some manner. The more you think about it, the more frightening it becomes.

Symptoms of Fructose Malabsorption

Symptoms of FM include:
(Not all FMers experience all symptoms.)

- Stomach pain
- Flatulence (passing gas)
- Acid indigestion/heartburn/acid reflux
- Diarrhea/constipation
- Bloating/swelling–this occurs internally as well as externally–making breathing labored and blocking sinuses
- Burping
- Bad Breath
- Nausea/vomiting

Also associated with FM:

- Headaches/migraines
- Brain fog
- Chronic fatigue
- Depression/mood disorders
- Sugar cravings
- Inability to lose or gain weight
- Hemorrhoids
- Concentration difficulties
- Dark circles under eyes
- Lack of sense of smell
- Difficulty sleeping
- Achy legs/restless leg syndrome
- fibroid pain/fibromyalgia
- irritable bladder-frequency and urgency

- Rosacea

Studies have also shown the following to be associated with FM:

- Iron deficiency
- High triglycerides
- Folic acid deficiency
- Elevated LDL cholesterol
- Zinc deficiency

With the exception of iron (which for me is on the low end of normal) and folic acid, (of which I am unaware) every item listed here described me. Learning of this condition and researching it has provided answers to many questions. The "treatment" brought both relief and other problems.

Diagnosis

A diagnosis of FM is done by a simple breath hydrogen test. This test is specific for fructose. There are other breath hydrogen tests, but only a fructose breath hydrogen test will test for FM. After fasting for eight to twelve hours, the patient begins the test by blowing into a small bag, which is then sealed, for a baseline sample, followed by drinking a solution of fructose water. The patient will then continue the process of blowing into a new small bag every twenty minutes for a period of time from two to five hours. I did this for three hours. After completion of the test, the bags are sent to the lab for analysis.

This test can also be done using a machine which will give immediate results, though few doctors have it available, while the bag version is inexpensive and readily available for any doctor's office to administer.

The patient is considered to have FM if the hydrogen levels in the samples are twenty points or more above the baseline sample level in two or more samples. My highest reading was 116. This test is simple and non-invasive, with its only negatives being the amount of time involved and the reaction to the fructose for those with FM.

Sample	Time	Clock	ppm H2
Baseline	0	8:35	0
1	20 minutes	8:55	0

2	40 minutes	9:15	29
3	1 hour	9:35	116
4	80 minutes	9:55	47
5	100 minutes	10:15	38
6	2 hours	10:35	36
7	140 minutes	10:55	57
8	160 minutes	11:15	29
9	3 hours	11:35	9

Copy of my Breath Hydrogen Test Results

Caution: Anyone suspected of having Hereditary Fructose Intolerance (HFI) should not have a fructose breath hydrogen test before undergoing tests for HFI since this could result in a serious hypoglycemic reaction.

As a result of the nutritional and dietary challenges faced by an FMer, I am completely baffled as to why anyone would self-diagnose this condition and not have a breath hydrogen test done. Aside from the many serious conditions which may go undetected with an improper opinion of FM, this is not easy to live with. Get tested!

Remember, you are in charge of your body. If you suspect you have FM and your physician is resistant to testing, you are allowed to be insistent. Where would I be if I had accepted the prescribed laxatives and not insisted on a referral to a gastroenterologist? The diet for FM is too life-changing to accept an opinion of FM without testing. So be insistent.

Some physicians are reluctant to order a breath hydrogen test because of the possibility of false positives or negatives. In the end, the decision is yours.

One of the difficulties in diagnosing FM without a breath hydrogen test is the vast array of seemingly unrelated symptoms. Additional complications arise when one considers that different foods trigger different symptoms.

While one food may produce the classic stomach cramps, another initiates puffiness. Though I am reluctant to repeat myself, I will—get tested.

Treatment for Fructose Malabsorption

The good news: There are no medications to take, surgery involved, or repeated visits to the doctor. The bad news: FM is treated by dietary restrictions. Unlike individuals who are lactose intolerant, FMers do not have the option of taking an enzyme to alleviate their condition. Lactose is a disaccharide (two sugar molecules), allowing those who are intolerant to take an enzyme to further break it down to a mono-saccharide (one sugar molecule), thus rendering it absorbable. However, fructose is a mono-saccharide, so it cannot be broken down further by taking an enzyme or any other medication. It is already at its basic form.

Fortunately, there is now far more information available on FM and its diet than when I was first diagnosed. Books, articles, groups, and internet information can now be found.

When I was first diagnosed, so few people were familiar with FM that it was difficult to find a dietician or nutritionist qualified to help. Even now, take care when searching for a dietician or nutritionist. Interview them before making an appointment. Ask how many clients they have worked with who have FM. In 2007, I spent seventy dollars for a consultation with a nutritionist—only to discover she knew less than I did. When I made the appointment, I asked if she was familiar with FM and received an affirmative answer. During our consultation, she used the same printouts I had gotten from researching FM on the internet. She appeared not to know the difference

14

between FM and HFI. After asking how many clients she had with FM, I discovered I was the first, and her familiarity with FM came from her conversation with the person who had referred me to her.

The gastroenterologist's nurse practitioner suggested I begin with at least two weeks of a totally fructose-free diet and gave me a small amount of information on the diet for HFI, which I had already found on the internet. This diet is very difficult. It does not allow any fructose or sugar. Reading labels proved this came close to a diet restricted to unprocessed meats, dairy, and fresh produce—most of which cannot be eaten.

I stayed on this diet for about six weeks hoping the extra time would allow my body to heal from some of what I had been through. Then I slowly added foods to see what I could tolerate.

A surprising advantage of this restriction came in the form of a relatively flat tummy. I had been wondering why I had gained so much in the entire stomach area, especially just below my bra. I had a "shelf" which distended out about two inches. Not only did my "shelf" go away, but so did the bulge on down my torso. I felt skinny. It was as though I had lost ten pounds. This result only took about a week. It was not weight; it was bloat.

The wonderful thing about living with FM is—after eating right for a short time—the symptoms disappear. The length of time seems to differ for each FMer (usually three days to two weeks). No waking in the middle of the night suffering from gas pains, no constipation/diarrhea, no foggy brain, no migraines/headaches. You get the idea. This is an amazing detail for a person who has lived with multiple,

15

seemingly unrelated, symptoms. Not only does it feel wonderful physically, but the mental and emotional relief involved is reassuring. Despite what some speculated, I am *not* a hypochondriac!

SIBO

Often coupled with FM is small intestine bacterial overgrowth (SIBO), which is exactly what it sounds like. The bacteria in the small intestine have multiplied to excessive quantities, which cause symptoms similar to FM. How does this multiplication of bacteria occur? There are several possibilities.

- Slow digestive system movement
- Problems with the ileocecal valve, located between the ileum (the end of the small intestine) and the cecum (the pouch forming the beginning of the large intestine). This valve prevents contents in the large intestine from backing up into the small intestine.
- Low stomach acid. Stomach acid is essential in breaking down food for digestion. When food is not sufficiently broken down before entering the small bowel, it provides extra food for the bacteria residing there, which results in a multiplication of bacteria. Additionally, gastric acid suppresses the growth of bacteria. Low stomach acid looks and feels like excessive stomach acid, resulting in the consumption of antacids and protein pump inhibitors (PPIs), which will exacerbate the low acid problem.
- Physical abnormalities of the digestive tract, such as scarring from surgery or illness.
- A weakened immune system

- A diet high in sugars, refined carbs, and alcohol.

What are the risk factors for SIBO?

- Low stomach acid
- IBS
- Celiac
- Crohn's disease
- Diabetes
- Prior bowel surgery
- Multiple courses of antibiotics
- Liver, pancreas, or kidney problems
- Alcohol consumption
- Oral birth control
- A diet high in sugars and carbs

What are the symptoms of SIBO?

- The same as the symptoms of FM

It is estimated that up to fifteen percent of people who show no symptoms have SIBO. But for those of us with FM or some form of IBS, that percentage increases to an estimated eighty percent. How is SIBO diagnosed? The primary diagnostic tool for SIBO is either a lactulose breath test or a glucose breath test, though the lactulose breath test is considered the gold standard. Note: this is different than a lactose breath test.

Because this is a hydrogen breath test, if it does not also test for methane, you may get a false negative. If you produce large amounts of methane, it can reduce hydrogen levels, resulting in a false negative. High methane is associated with constipation. Those treated for SIBO show an improvement in regularity. Because methane leads to increased production of short-chain fatty acids, it has been linked to obesity and high BMIs.

How is SIBO treated? The answer to this question sounds better than the one for treating FM. It depends on your point of view and how you decide to treat it. Some lean toward an aggressive approach, using antibiotics specifically designed to attack the gut. Others decide on a slower, more natural approach to treatment.

Antibiotics

While most antibiotics travel throughout the body, with only about ten percent remaining in the gut, almost all of Xifaxan and Neomyacin remain in the digestive system. This makes both drugs good options for treating SIBO. However, they both have disadvantages.

Xifaxan (also known as rifaximin) is currently very expensive ($600-$1000 per round), with no generics available as of this writing. It's possible your gastroenterologist may have samples to provide for a full round. This is especially important because not all insurance companies will cover Xifaxan for treatment of SIBO.

Neomycin is much less expensive but is associated with many problematic side effects, causing some gastros to hesitate to prescribe it.

Antibiotics will lead to quick and complete relief. However, they must be accompanied by diet changes or SIBO will return.

Herbal Antibiotics

One study supported the use of enteric-coated peppermint oil for twenty days with a success rate of twenty-five to fifty percent.

Microb Clear™, a blend of magnesiumcaprylate, berberine, and extracts from tribulus, sweet wormwood,

19

grapefruit, barberry, bearberry, and black walnut produced by Amy Myers, MD, is purported to kill bacteria naturally.

Herbal remedies can interact with other medications, so be sure to check with your doctor before trying.

Diet

While adjustments to your diet will be necessary to keep SIBO from returning, it may also be eliminated by diet alone. The problem is, it is a long-term project, and does not offer immediate relief of symptoms.

If you choose to go the diet route, you will need to eliminate all sugars and carbs from your diet for an extended period.

Regardless of which healing route you choose, you will need to limit the foods that feed the bacteria to prevent a reoccurrence: sugar, carbs, alcohol…

Despite my determination to use antibiotics only when absolutely necessary, I chose the antibiotic route. By the time I discovered I also had SIBO, almost anything I ate made me ill. (The current knowledge regarding SIBO came years after my FM diagnosis, so no mention was made of it until I returned to the gastro requesting to be tested.)

Leaky Gut

Leaky gut may sound like a made-up condition, but it is being recognized by more and more professionals. The more you learn about it, the more it makes sense.

Also known as intestinal permeability, increased intestinal permeability, or hyperpermeable intestines, leaky gut occurs when the intestinal lining is compromised. The small intestine is about twenty feet long, with a surface area equal to a tennis court. The primary function of the small intestine is the absorption of nutrients and minerals from food. Small, finger-like protrusions, villi, are responsible for absorption. The wall of the small intestine is thin, sticking together with tight junctions. When compromised, these tight junctions can break, wreaking havoc.

LEAKY GUT

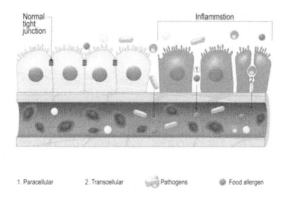

Normal tight junction   Inflammstion

1. Paracellular   2. Transcellular   Pathogens   Food allergen

This allows incompletely digested particles into the bloodstream. These particles may include nutrients, toxins, and bacteria. Things that should be pooped out are entering the body.

Hippocrates said, "All disease begins in the gut." Since leaky gut is associated with many diseases, including FM, IBS, fibroid pain, autoimmune diseases, chronic fatigue, ADHD, allergies, acne, etc., I would say he was wise.

The symptoms of leaky gut are the same as for FM, with potential additional symptoms: respiratory problems, such as asthma; behavioral problems, such as ADHD; fertility problems; adrenal fatigue; and liver problems.

How does leaky gut happen? Inflammation, poor diet, NSAID use, gluten, SIBO, gastrointestinal infections, alcohol, smoking, caffeinated drinks, soda, chocolate, processed foods, antibiotics (including those in meats), and stress are all associated with leaky gut.

If you have a form of IBS, FM included, you can assume you have leaky gut. However, if you prefer to know for sure, there is a test, the lactulose-mannitol test. (Be forewarned, many tradition MDs still do not recognize leaky gut.) After drinking a small amount of lactulose-mannitol, urine samples will be collected for five to six hours. The mannitol is tiny and should show up in the urine. The lactulose should not be able to permeate the intestinal wall, allowing it to be pooped out. If it has permeated the intestinal wall, the body cannot use lactulose, so the kidneys will eliminate it in urine.

Can leaky gut be cured or improved? Yes. Once again, this involves diet.

- Avoid foods which cause a reaction.
- Avoid refined vegetable oils, refined sugars and artificial sweeteners, gluten, and grains
- Treat SIBO infections

- Consume homemade bone broth (should have a gelatin consistency when cold), sprouted seeds, coconut products, fermented vegetables, and apple cider vinegar

When I first learned of leaky gut, I was reacting to almost everything I ate. With time and care (see above), I can now eat a wide variety of foods without problems. There are easy to understand articles with excellent illustrations:

- https://examinedexistence.com/leaky-gut-syndrome-fix/
- https://healthygut.com/articles/the-scd-diet-and-leaky-gut-syndrome/

If you don't want to make your own bone broth, I've found two without added onions, Pure Bone Broth, by Au Bon and Turmeric Chicken Bone Broth, by Nona Lim. Both are available on Amazon.

Poop

Yes, we have a chapter on poop. Why? If we've always pooped the same way, we may not understand we are not normal.

For instance, I always pooped once a week or less, straining as I did so. I had no idea this was not normal. After all, it was normal for me. But I was constipated.

What is normal? The following is designed to help you determine what you are.

- Rabbit Pellets: round, hard, individual stools that are difficult to expel
- Lumpy Log: can see round stools joined into one lumpy log that is difficult to expel
- Sausage Shaped: shaped like a sausage with possible cracks on the surface and is easy to expel
- Sausage: smooth sausage shape that is easy to expel
- Blobs: soft, individual blobs that are easy to expel
- Mush: large, soft pile that is easy to expel
- Liquid: liquid and very easy to expel

So what is normal? Sausage Shaped or Sausage.

If you have rabbit pellets, a lumpy log, or need to strain to go, you are constipated.

If you have blobs, mush, or liquid, you have diarrhea. Don't stop looking yet.

- Floating Poop: fatty poop, too much fat or unable to digest and absorb fat properly

- Food Particles: poop laced with pieces of food, need to chew more or have low stomach acid

The good news is, once your diet is good, your poop will be too.

The Diet

Due to the nature of food intolerances, different people have different levels of tolerance to offensive foods. While some cannot tolerate any, others react only to large quantities. This makes a defined diet difficult. Ask ten different FMers, and you will receive ten different lists of foods. However, all ten lists will also have many basic common foods.

Most fruits and vegetables contain a mixture of fructose and glucose. According to research,[1] it is the ratio of this mixture, restricted to fructose never higher than glucose, which the FMer needs to be concerned.

"Absorption is enhanced by co-ingestion with glucose, since glucose uptake stimulates additional transport pathways for fructose absorption in the small intestinal epithelial cell."[1]

As a result,

"People with fructose malabsorption need to avoid foods high in free fructose, but can manage those with balanced concentrations of fructose and glucose (or a greater concentration of glucose)."[1]

When fructose is higher than glucose, it is referred to as free fructose. As a way of proving this theory,

"19 patients with an abnormal breath test and symptoms following fructose were reexamined after a load with equimolar concentrations of glucose and fructose. Hydrogen breath test was normal in all of them, none developed abdominal discomfort."[3]

This fructose-glucose ratio component reveals that FMers can eat some fruits, but only in limited quantities.

"In addition to excess fructose foods, those high in the balanced sugars may also be problematic when consumed in large amounts as these provide a high fructose load. For example, an orange is in equal balance of fructose and glucose so is safe to eat, however, orange juice is concentrated, with one glass containing up to six oranges, so this should be limited to only one-third glass in one sitting (equivalent to the juice from one serving of fruit)."[1]

In other words, be sure the balance of fructose to glucose is higher in glucose, and then limit the quantity.

When I first discovered this, it had been a year since I had consumed any fruit. The ratio idea made perfect sense to me since citrus fruits have been the only fruit I had ever eaten which helped to loosen my digestive system.

After learning I might be able to eat an orange, I tried half of a small one. That first bite was amazing! It was as though I had bitten into a juicy, flavorful piece of heaven. I closed my eyes and savored every nuance of it: from the glorious aroma, to the beady texture, to the luscious juiciness, to the explosive flavor. Eating that orange was a definite pinnacle of dining experiences. Chocolate never tasted that good. Even better, there was no reaction.

An exception to the fructose-glucose ratio is found in foods containing polyols, of which sorbitol is the most common. Maltitol and isomalt are also types of polyols.

"Their absorption is not accelerated by co-ingestion with glucose but seems to be worse when given concomitantly with glucose."[1]

Sorbitol is an alternative sweetener commonly used in diabetic foods. Polyols are also added to chewing gum to

27

prevent tooth decay because they are not broken down by the bacteria in the mouth as sugar is. Unfortunately, it is also found in "stone" fruits, such as plums, apricots, and cherries. Consequently, despite the favorable ratio of these fruits, they are not normally appropriate for those with FM.

Wheat is another problem with FM.

"A person can suffer from wheat intolerance but not fructose malabsorption. However, if they have fructose malabsorption, they will have problems with high intakes of wheat."[6]

However,

"Wheat is a problem in large amounts, i.e., when it is the main ingredient in a product."[1]

Hence, bread, pasta, and pastries may be problematic for those with FM.

Why is wheat not safe? Wheat is in the fructan category. Technically, these are chains of fructose molecules ending with a glucose molecule. In English, they allow the plant to thrive in low temperatures and during drought. Though tolerance for fructans varies, they are not usually acceptable for FMers. Wheat, spelt, barley, brown rice (the hull of the rice), onions, and garlic, are a few of the fructans to avoid.

At first, I discovered it was best for me to stay away from the whole-wheat variety of pasta and breads. Limiting the quantity I ate also helped. Rather than having a whole sandwich, I limited myself to one-half a sandwich. Since then, I discovered I react far more to fructans than fructose. While I can sometimes tolerate small amounts of fructose, even a tiny amount of fructans cause problems. Since switching to gluten-free (gluten-containing foods also contain fructans) and fructan-free (no onions, garlic, etc.), I have been symptom-free.

Quantity restriction is important for those with FM. In addition to eating limited amounts of foods with a "glucose higher than fructose" ratio, quantity, in general, should be limited. In the digestive tract,

"the contents comprise solid, liquid and gas components and dietary factors can influence all of these."[1]

The conclusion may then be drawn that, since it is difficult for the FM sufferer to avoid problematic foods entirely and there is limited capacity within the digestive tract, larger quantities of food coupled with liquid and gas will be more likely to result in pain.

I have found the above to be quite accurate. So much so that for a while I restricted myself to six mini-meals rather than large meals, regardless of what I ate. It helped some. Since discovering fructans were most of my problem, I have gone back to three main meals, or even two, with no problem. But I have never been a big eater.

Also, an FMer must consider their "bucket." This is the little bits of offending foods you've eaten in recent days that in large quantity may cause a reaction but in small quantity does not. For example, Sunday you eat a little green pepper without a reaction. Monday you have a small apple with no reaction. Tuesday morning, you have three cherries with no reaction. Tuesday evening, you eat a couple sticks of celery. That night you awaken in pain. Each day's consumption by itself was not a problem. However, when added together in your bucket, the bucket overflowed Tuesday night, causing a reaction. As FMers, we must always be conscious of our buckets.

Thankfully, we now have the FODMAP diet. This is available in book form or app form. A result of research by a Monash University (Australia) team, the FODMAP diet provides guidance not previously available to FMers.

For a small fee, the Monash University Low FODMAP diet™ app is available. In addition to a food guide, it includes recipes, an IBS explanation booklet, a diary, dietitian training, and a list of certified FODMAP companies (many in Australia). The food is listed by category (vegetables, fruit, beverages, etc.), and rated with a red/yellow/green stoplight system, and includes information on why it is rated as it is. For processed foods, the app also includes flags telling what countries the products are available. Their continued research makes this the most up-to-date, extensive, and reliable list available.

Also available are free FODMAP apps. One is Fast FODMAP. It allows the user to enter the food in question; then it shows a red/yellow/green rectangle with an explanation of what the problem is. The app also includes a learning game and a diary.

The apps I've seen give serving amounts. Larger servings may not be acceptable, even if a food is acceptable.

One more note on apps, they may sometimes disagree with each other. At this writing, Monash is considered the most reliable.

Sugars & Sweeteners

There are many different types of sugar, each from different sources, with different possible consequences for the FMer.

I believe the reason my FM problem became so acute, necessitating diagnosis, is when we ran out of table sugar at work I discovered Splenda® and began using it instead of sugar. Splenda® and FM do not get along.

As with most foods, each FMer must determine which sugars they can tolerate and to what extent. For instance, I enjoy rare use of organic cane sugar, which has a 50:50 ratio of fructose/glucose, but as with all sugars, quantities must be limited. It is my understanding many FMers cannot tolerate even small quantities of table sugar. As the table below will reveal, this may be due to eating table sugar made with beet sugar rather than cane sugar.

I frequently have people ask me if I have to follow a diabetic diet. The answer–absolutely not. Diabetics must restrict their intake of glucose, thus a frequent substitute for sugar in their diets is sorbitol. Conversely, the FMer must avoid sorbitol completely and requires an appropriate fructose/glucose ratio (with glucose being higher). Hence, our diets are not even closely related. If you are a diabetic and an FMer, work with your dietician.

Be careful about foods which are "sugar-free." They frequently contain artificial sweeteners. Also be cautious with foods labeled "fat-free" or "low fat," which frequently add sugar or artificial sweeteners to compensate for the loss of fat. As always, read the labels.

The following chart is an adaptation of the "Sugars & Sweeteners" chart on the Boston University website for hereditary fructose intolerance (HFI)[11] (Used by permission). The original chart includes a wide variety of sugars and sweeteners which are not common and for those of us hoping to simplify and understand, can be rather overwhelming, so we have provided this condensed version listing the more common sweeteners. Additionally, the original chart was designed for HFI patients (thus resulting in more confusion for the FMer). We have revised it for the FMer. The tolerance column has been changed to reflect FMers tolerance as gleaned from my experience, coupled with comments from other FMers. Remember, tolerance levels may differ, and quantity is a factor. Determine your own tolerance levels. The "?" in the tolerance column is an indication that tolerance seems to vary widely.

Sugar Sweetener	Description	Tolerance
Agave Syrup	From the blue agave cactus. Commonly used in Tex-Mex foods, tequila, margaritas, soft drinks. High in fructose.	No

Aspartame	Sugar substitute known as Equal, NutraSweet, NutraTase. FDA approved. Scientifically studied in depth. Some may be sensitive to headaches. Derived from amino acids. Be aware-there are many non-FM negative effects to aspartame.	Yes
Barley Malt Syrup	From sprouted grains of barley, kiln dried and cooked with water.	No
Beet Sugar	Sucrose. Same structure as cane sugar, but may produce different product results because of .05 differences in minerals and proteins. More common in Europe than the U.S. Often cheap brands in US.	No
Brown Rice Syrup	Made from brown rice. High protein content. Likely contains sucrose.	?
Brown Sugar	Sucrose coated with molasses.	Yes
Cane Sugar	Sucrose. Table sugar.	Yes
Corn Starch	Derived from corn. Composed of straight or branched chains of glucose.	Yes

Corn Sugar	Produced from corn starch. Contains glucose and maltose molecules.	Yes
Corn Syrup	Glucose and water. Usually produced from cornstarch. The problem is that in making the syrup, it may have either maltose and/or fructose added.	Yes
Corn Syrup Solids	Dried glucose syrup.	Yes
Confectioners Sugar	Sucrose. A chemical combination of glucose and fructose.	Yes
Date Sugar	Made from dried, pulverized dates. Likely contains sucrose.	? No
Dextrin	Glucose molecules linked together in chains. Does not break down to pure dextrose.	Yes
Dextrose	Single glucose molecule. Simple sugar.	Yes

Evaporated Cane Sugar	Sucrose. Another name for sugar cane juice.	Yes
Fructose	Simple sugar of fructose molecules. Sometimes called fruit sugar. Made of 6 carbons.	No
Fruit Juice Sweeteners	Derived from grapes, apples or pears, heated to reduce water leaving a sweeter more concentrated juice. Almost pure fructose.	No
Glucose	Simple sugar. The chemical sugar structure of blood sugar. Made of 6 carbons.	Yes
Granulated sugar	Table sugar. Sucrose. Can be tolerated only if it is pure cane sugar, not beet sugar.	Yes
High Fructose Corn Syrup (HFCS)	Enzymetically converted from corn syrup to contain 42% - 90% fructose. Raises triglyceride levels and may increase risk of heart disease. See the chapter on HFCS.	No
Honey	Natural syrup containing about 35% glucose, 40% fructose, 25 % water	No

Inverted Sugar	Created by combining sugar syrup with cream of tarter or lemon juice and heating, breaking sucrose down to components glucose and fructose.	No
Isoglucose	Another name for High Fructose Corn Syrup (HFCS).	No
Isomalt	Polyol	No
Levulose	Contains fructose.	No
Maltitol	Sugar alcohol form of maltose (glucose). This is a polyol.	No
Maltose	Linked glucose molecules that rapidly break down to glucose in the intestine.	Yes
Maple Syrup	Mostly sucrose. Only 100% Pure.	Yes

Molasses	By-product of sugar cane with 24% water. Fructose level varies. Three kinds. Light (sweetest), Medium (darker and less sweet), Blackstrap (very dark, slightly sweet with distinctive flavor. Good source of calcium and iron.) Also contains fructans.	No
Molasses Sugar	Dark muscovado sugar with extra molasses.	No
Raffinose	A trisaccharide found in grains, legumes and some vegetables. Gas forming.	No
Raw Sugar	Sucrose. Equal parts glucose and fructose, a chemical combination of glucose and fructose.	Yes
Saccharin	Sugar substitute. Not as commonly used as in the past. Known as Sweet N' Low, Sugar Twin, Sucryl, Featherweight. FDA approved. More than 6 servings per day may increase bladder cancer risk. (No longer approved for use in Canada)	No
Sorbitol	Sugar alcohol. Common in fruits, particularly skin of ripe berries, cherries and plums. Used in sugar free foods. Causes diarrhea. Converted back to fructose. This is a polyol.	No

Splenda	A sugar substitute. This is a chemically modified sucrose molecule that cannot be digested.	No
Stevia	Natural sweetener from a South American plant. 30 % sweeter than sugar. Used extensively in Japan, China, Korea, Israel, Brazil and Paraguay with no side effects reported. Known as Stevioside. Has not been rigorously tested for safety. No consistent manufacturing regulations.	Yes
Sucralose	Chemical name for Splenda, a sugar substitute. Large molecule not digested.	No
Sucrose	Naturally occurring sugar made from sugar cane or sugar beets. Commonly referred to as sugar and table sugar. Chemical combination of glucose and fructose. Tolerated if from cane but not from beets.	Yes
Sucrose Syrups	Also known as Refiner's syrup. By product of sugar refining. 18% water, 1 part sucrose to two parts invert sugar. Invert sugar turns to fructose when eaten.	No
Sugar	Common name for sucrose, a chemical combination of glucose and fructose.	Yes

Xylitol	Sugar alcohol. Obtained from fruits and berries. Also from birch trees and known as birch sugar. May causes diarrhea.	No

High Fructose Corn Syrup

Read a few labels next time you go to the grocery store. There is a very good chance you will see high fructose corn syrup (HFCS) on most of them. In the United States, it is in the soda you drink, many canned fruits, cereal, yogurt, bread, peanut butter, ketchup, the list goes on and on. Thankfully, due to consumer awareness, more and more products are eliminating HFCS.

Technically, HFCS is

"enzyme-catalyzed isomerization of glucose (dextrose) to the sweeter sugar, fructose (levulose)."[2]

Stated in somewhat more comprehensible English:

"undergone enzymatic processing in order to increase their fructose content and are then mixed with pure corn syrup (100% glucose)"[4]

Unfortunately,

"Subsequent development of separation processes for enriching the fructose content not only allowed production of syrups with higher fructose content than could be produced by enzymatic action alone, but ultimately allowed the manufacture of pure crystalline fructose from starch."[2]

HFCS was developed in 1957, refined in the 1970s, and began a rapid introduction to foods from 1975 to 1985 (see charts at the end of this chapter).

One source we initially found actually listed HFCS as acceptable for those with FM.

"HFCS is made up of almost half glucose and half fructose and may be absorbed just as well as sucrose (regular table sugar)"[7].

However, there are different types of HFCS:

40

HFCS 90 (most commonly used in baked goods), approximately 90% fructose and 10% glucose

HFCS 55 (most commonly used in soft drinks), approximately 55% fructose and 45% glucose

HFCS 42 (most commonly used in sports drinks), approximately 42% fructose and 58% glucose [4]

As it is easy to see, only one of these falls within the 50% or less fructose limit. Foods containing HFCS do not state which HFCS the food contains, so we have no way of determining for sure if the glucose is greater than the fructose. The University of Virginia resource is the only one I have found which said HFCS is acceptable. All others warn against its use. My experience also indicates it is unacceptable for FM sufferers. A perusal of FM internet support sites shows other FMers also find it unacceptable.

Though controversial, many believe, and studies have shown, HFCS to be linked to various health problems, including obesity, heart disease, and diabetes. According to the Nutritional Research Center.Org,

"In 2005, if one looks at the actuarial curve on cardiovascular disease, obesity, hypoglycemia, and diabetes, they all parallel HFCS increase in the food chain—A FACT."

Think about it. In the mid-1980s, the health-conscious movement began. Aerobics, gyms, running, and other forms of exercise became the norm. The contradiction in these two facts tells me there is at least one major contributing factor. I believe it to be HFCS.

According to Satish Rao, M.D., of the University of Iowa, though we have long consumed fructose in the form of fruits,

"...what has changed in recent decades is that many people in the United States eat vastly more fructose and in a purer form rather than mixed with other sugars." (HFCS)

This leads me to the assumption that the super concentration of fructose I used to ingest in the form of HFCS may have been detrimental to my health.

As with everything in this book, you must form your own opinion about HFCS and make your own decisions.

Obesity rates from 1960 to 2000

Overweight and obesity

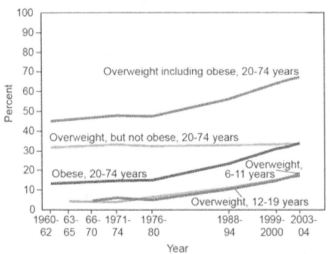

SOURCES: Centers for Disease Control and Prevention, National Center for Health Statistics, Health, United States, 2006. Figure 13. Data from the National Health and Nutrition Examination Survey

According to the National Center for Health (NCH), average weight has increased, with obesity rates now at record levels. Between 1962 and 2000, obese people grew from 13% to 31% of the population. According to the NCH, one-third of U.S. adults, or over 72 million people, were obese in 2005-2006. The dictionary defines obese as having a body weight more than 20 percent greater than recommended for the relevant height.

42

Obesity rates from 2000 to 2016

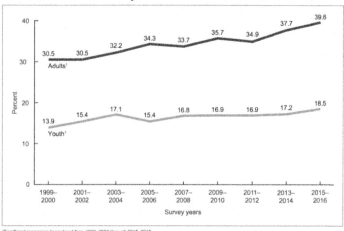

'Significant increasing linear trend from 1999–2000 through 2015–2016.
NOTES: All estimates for adults are age adjusted by the direct method to the 2000 U.S. census population using the age groups 20–39, 40–59, and 60 and over.
Access data table for Figure 5 at: https://www.cdc.gov/nchs/data/databriefs/db288_table.pdf#5.
SOURCE: NCHS, National Health and Nutrition Examination Survey, 1999–2016.

Adult obesity rates, 1990 to 2017

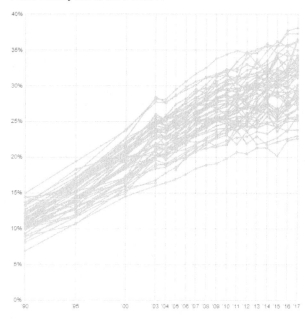

1. Obesity rates in each US state. www.stateofobesity.org/adult-obesity/

As you can see from the graphs, obesity in adults has risen from 13% in 1960 to 39.6% in 2016. Note in the first figure, the obesity, overweight, and children's overweight rates remained stable until a steady rise in rates commenced in 1976-1980.

"The latest federal data show that nearly 40 percent of American adults were obese in 2015–16, up from 34 percent in 2007–08... In 1985, no state had an obesity rate higher than 15 percent. In 2016, five states had rates over 35 percent."[14]

All this happens to coincide with the rapid introduction of HFCS into foods. Coincidence or results?

What *Can* I Eat?

Good question. When I was diagnosed, this is where the conflicting information really started. One source said a food is acceptable while another said never eat it. For example, early on, my husband spent an entire afternoon comparing the six lists we had at that time for acceptable foods. Since I was still having problems, despite a strict diet, he was hoping to discover a "for sure" list of foods I could eat. Of the six lists compared, there were five vegetables found on all six as acceptable. Of those five, my current research has shown several to be potentially unacceptable. So what is the FM sufferer to do?

This is the list Bob compiled of foods which are on all six lists as acceptable foods. Do not use it.

Protein	Veggies	Dairy	Breads & Cereals	Carbs
Beef	Asparagus	Milk	Ezekiel Bread	
				Potatoes
Pork	Peppers	Cheese	Sprouted Grain Bread	
				Pasta
Chicken	Cauliflower	Butter	Unsweetened bread	
Turkey	Celery	Sour Cream	Oatmeal	
Venison	Spinach	Unsweetened Yogurt	White Rice	
Fish	Mushrooms			
Nuts				
Tofu				
Eggs				
Seafood				

First and foremost, educate yourself. Rather than writing a book of "dos and don'ts," we have tried to provide a source which will give you the reasoning behind the dos and don'ts, such as why to stay away from stone fruits (polyols) when some sources say they are fine due to their

45

fructose/glucose ratio. Hopefully, this will help you wade through some of the conflicting information.

In our first edition, we recommended you begin with a sugar-free, fructose-free diet for a minimum of two weeks. This is the diet for HFI. I stuck with it for about six weeks before beginning to add foods in hopes of giving some extra relief to my taxed body. Thankfully, the low-FODMAP diet is now available.

FODMAP is an acronym for Fermentable Oligosaccharides, Disaccharides, Monosaccharides and Polyols. Notice four of these items end with saccharides? Saccharides are sugars. These FODMAPs are resistant to digestion. Most foods would be absorbed into your bloodstream in the small intestine to feed your body, but theses sugary FODMAPs remain in your digestive system, reaching your large intestine where they feed the large number of bacteria residing there. The by-product of these bacteria is hydrogen, which causes gas, bloating, pain, and constipation. Because FODMAPs are osmotic, they can also draw water, causing diarrhea.

FODMAPs are found in foods such as:

Fructose: fruits, vegetables, honey, HFCS

Fructans: onions, leeks, garlic, artichokes, wheat, barley, rye

Galacto-Oligosaccharides (GOS): legumes (pinto beans, kidney beans), lentils, chickpeas

Lactose: milk and other dairy products including soft cheeses

Polyols: stone fruits, such as plums, sweeteners ending in ol, such as mannitol and xylitol

The low-FODMAP diet was developed by a research group at Monash University in Melbourne, Australia. The researchers at Monash have tested and rated many foods for

FODMAPs. Foods are rated high, medium, or low, with low being the safe foods.

For a list of FODMAPS, turn to page 128. If you have a smartphone, you can download one of several available FODMAP apps. Many are free. This will give you an on-the-go resource.

Sue Shepherd, Ph.D., one of the Monash researchers, recommends a strict restriction of all FODMAPs for four to six weeks. Apparently, I was wise in my length of restriction.

Adding foods must be done slowly, one at a time. The most difficult part of adding foods is, when a food disagrees with you, you need to wait several days to two weeks, to allow the body to return to normal before trying a new food. It is a long process which takes a great deal of patience.

Food diaries are highly recommended. Both the free Fast FODMAP app and the Monash app I have installed on my smartphone also includes an extensive food diary tab which allows you to record emotional and physical wellness, where you ate, and what you ate.

When you begin adding new foods, I recommend you add them from one category. For instance, if you think you can tolerate lactose, add foods that contain lactose first. This was how I finally determined that what I react to most are fructans.

When I began my FM journey, there was a great deal of misinformation available on the internet and no books. We were left with discernment and trial and error. Learning about the fructose/glucose ratio was helpful but still conflicting. The Monash University team and their low-FODMAP diet have made food questions much easier for us and our loved ones.

When shopping–this cannot be said enough–read labels. An excellent example of the label being the FMers friend is yogurt. Many popular yogurts have HFCS. Many organic varieties contain molasses or honey. Both these items are high FODMAP. But do not despair, safe yogurts do exist. Even if you are lactose sensitive. We just have to look harder for them. Most will contain cane sugar; be sure you can handle small amounts before trying yogurt.

If you are accustomed to eating out frequently or eating boxed, frozen, or pre-prepared foods, be prepared to change. Learn to cook from scratch. Whole foods are not only healthier but easier for the FMer to discern acceptability than prepared and processed foods. Plus, there are no lists of ingredients to read through.

Don't be afraid to adjust recipes to fit your individual needs. For instance, you can leave onions and garlic out of recipes. If you miss them, you may want to add small amounts of asafetida powder. One note on asafetida, whatever you do, don't taste it raw. It's vile tasting!

Unfortunately, there are no "Safe for FM" or "FODMAP Safe" labels required on foods—yet. Nor are nutrition labels required to divide the "sugars" into the types of sugars (fructose, glucose, sucrose, etc.), allowing us to determine the fructose/glucose ratio—yet. Perhaps as FM becomes better known and the numbers of diagnosed FMers increase, such labeling will be a reality. Until recently, "Gluten Free" labeling did not exist.

Ultimately, each FMer must customize their individual diet. Make your own lists of yes, no, and maybe foods. As an aid, we have provided lists in the appendix of this book. See page 128. These lists are not set in stone, add to them as you learn. Additionally, there may be foods which can only be eaten in combination with other foods or in small quantities.

Remember, regardless if a list in this book or on a website says a certain food is okay, you cannot make the assumption it is okay for you until you are able to eat it symptom-free on a consistent basis. Educate yourself and those around you. This is not an overnight process. But thanks to the researchers at Monash University, it is much faster and we no longer need to feel like lab rats.

Nutrition Notes

As stated earlier, I have long been a nutrition-conscious person, especially with my children. I find it amusing that recently there has been a great deal of hype regarding colors of foods in our diets. It seems either the media or the health experts have just figured out that the greater the variety of natural colors in our diets, the more vitamins and minerals we will get, thus resulting in healthier bodies. By colors I refer to the dark green of spinach, Swiss chard, or broccoli; the orange of carrots, oranges, or yams; the red of cherries, tomatoes, or beets; the yellow of peaches, corn, or squash; the white of cauliflower, potatoes, or onions, etc.

My now grown children will tell you this is something I have stressed since they were small. As the old saying goes, "Variety is the spice of life." In my way of thinking, this refers to food. Unfortunately, this variety can be quite difficult for an FMer to achieve. Even when we can include a color, it is often necessary to restrict the quantity to such a small amount, we wonder how many benefits we are receiving. The FODMAP diet has made this much easier for FMers.

It has always been my opinion that if a person eats a good, nutritious diet, consisting of a wide variety of healthy foods, supplements should not be necessary. Unfortunately, few people these days seem to fit into this category. For the FMer, we need to be even more conscience of this need.

In addition to remaining conscious of the variety in my diet, we take a good quality multi-vitamin. This was also encouraged by my physician.

Supplements with inulin and fructooligosaccharide (FOS), both types of fructans, should be avoided. (Inulin is also used to replace fat in low-fat foods, so beware.) While current FODMAP lists say cellulose is okay, I do not tolerate it at all. Since it is found in many vitamins/pills/foods, be aware of your reaction to it.

Finding a good vitamin in either capsule form or gel-cap form without it being a "mega-vitamin" with an excessive percentage of nutrients is not easy.

I stress either capsule or gel-cap forms because I want to be getting the most for my money. A quick study will show most pill form vitamins are compressed so tightly they do not have time to absorb into your system before passing on to your bowels, thus wasting the remainder of the pill. If a pill does not completely dissolve within ten minutes in a glass of water, it will also not dissolve within your system.

Probiotics have been a source of controversy among the FM community. Some say they may help, some say they are a waste of money, and yet others say they will make matters worse (too much bacteria already, why add to the mix?). One FMer said her dietician said to stay away from anything with them.

My thoughts are, they should not hurt anything, so I take one per day. Be aware; there are many different types of probiotics. One of them, the probiotic bacterium, *Lactobacillus plantarum* 299V, was found to be effective in reducing IBS symptoms.[10] Just be sure they do not contain inulins.

When I first began my research, I thought probiotics and prebiotics were terms used interchangeably. I have since learned that prebiotics are active mainly in the small intestine and probiotics work only within the large intestine. When used in combination, they are referred to as synbiotics.

Recently, I have added vitamin D_3 to the mix of supplements I take. After being told my vitamin D levels are low, I did a bit of research into its source, its benefits, and what the effects of too little can be.

The most plentiful source of vitamin D is the sun (the USBs produce D_3). Regrettably, many of us spend the vast majority of each day indoors, we live in areas where the sun is in short supply during the winter months, or we live in smoggy areas. When we do get outside, we use sunscreen to prevent skin cancer; unfortunately, the downside to increased use of sunscreen is it also blocks the body from absorbing this necessary vitamin. Skin pigment also plays a role in the amount of vitamin D absorbed by the skin; the darker the skin, the less easily the vitamin D absorbs.

Other sources are fish and fortified products, such as cereals and milk. The D vitamin obtained through food is D_2. Regrettably, it is difficult to acquire enough of this essential vitamin from food alone. See page 108 for a list of vitamin D sources.

Vitamin D deficiency can lead to or is associated with: autoimmune diseases such as multiple sclerosis and rheumatoid arthritis, diabetes, cardiovascular diseases, cancer, depression, fractures, high blood pressure, infectious diseases, muscle weakness, osteoporosis, and rickets. Pediatricians throughout the country have been seeing patients suffering from rickets, which was once thought of as a problem from previous times. Furthermore, studies have shown that sufferers of chronic pain frequently have low levels of vitamin D. Sufferers of restless leg syndrome have reported improvement upon supplementation with vitamin D.

While there is some controversy surrounding the recommended allowance of vitamin D, there is no doubt we need to be sure we are not deficient in this essential vitamin. Rather than supplementing your diet "just-in-case," I suggest you ask your doctor to check your levels of vitamin D. This is done with a simple blood test.

When taking a supplement of a single vitamin or mineral, it is important to be sure you need it or are not taking excess amounts. The vitamins and minerals in our bodies are a delicate balance. If one vitamin or mineral is low, we show symptoms. This is exampled by, with low vitamin D, we may have achy bones; with low vitamin C, we may incur excessive bruising. On the other end of the spectrum, if we are taking levels which are too high, we can create an imbalance of other vitamins and minerals, causing other symptoms. Multi-vitamins are formulated to allow for this balance. Before taking any single vitamin or any mega vitamins, check with your doctor.

My doctor ordered a saliva test which checked for deficiencies. The results came back in an easy-to-read form, allowing me to add the needed supplements to my regimen.

Remember also that it is important to include any vitamin, mineral, or herbal supplements on your list of medications taken when seeing your physician. Certain combinations of medications and supplements are inadvisable due to interactions, being rendered ineffective by their combination, or potential false results on tests. Also, before planned surgery, certain supplements need to be discontinued due to potential adverse effects.

Ultimately, FMers must be extra conscious of the nutritional value of their diets. I have found this to be something I must do on my own since I have been unable to locate a dietician who is familiar enough with FM to be of assistance; we live in a remote, small town. I still attempt to vary the color of my meals as much as possible, adding the supplements mentioned above. Though I may not be achieving the nutritional value I hope to, my body is obviously healthier and happier with this new eating lifestyle as evidenced by a reduction and/or elimination of symptoms previously mentioned.

Mourning

If you have been diagnosed with FM, it is important to recognize that you have suffered a loss, one which will change most people's lives dramatically. Your loved ones will also need to understand this. As with any major loss in life, you will go through a mourning period. *Let yourself mourn.* You have, in a sense, suffered a death; the death of a way of life, a way of eating, a way of socializing.

Allowing yourself to mourn does not mean giving in to the depression, anger, or denial you may be experiencing, but instead, being aware of it for what it is and realizing it is something you *can* get through.

As with mourning anything, there is a process with stages. Familiarizing yourself with these stages may help you to understand and therefore better cope with the process. I must emphasize, this too shall pass. You *can* get used to FM. You *can* learn how to eat. You *can* learn to accept your condition. You can even learn to handle food in social situations.

St*eps of Mourning*

1. Shock – This is rather self-describing. It is shocking to discover the "healthy" eating you have been doing is contributing to making you ill. It is shocking to learn how many foods you can no longer eat. It is shocking to learn what is included in so many foods you eat.

2. Denial – Your denial may be in the form of eating freely, which will result in a harsh reminder you are unable to do this. Or you may deny the

55

permanency of this condition. (I still have hope.) You may even choose to hide your condition from friends or family to avoid such things as questions, pity, and disbelief.

3. Anger – It is easy to get angry about this. Anger and denial seem to accompany each other frequently during this process. There is so much to be angry about, but there is also so much for which to be thankful. Try to focus on these. Early after my diagnosis, when I was quite angry and busy feeling sorry for myself, I realized I actually had it easy. I worked with three people who were battling cancer. For them, it was life or death. For them, treatment was agonizing. For them, merely having to restrict their diet would have been a relief. How dare I spend so much time and energy wallowing in self-pity? I was, and still am, ashamed of myself for this. When I begin to feel sorry for myself I try to remember my co-workers and others who have *real* problems.

4. Depression – Anger has a way of leading to self-pity; this, in turn, contributes to depression. To help you deal with depression, see the chapter on depression and seek professional help if needed.

5. Acceptance – From the First Edition—I am finally, after two years, at this point. Do I still have to deal with any of the aforementioned steps? You bet I do. I still get angry. I still wallow in self-pity and depression. I'm constantly testing the boundaries. I even still try denial at times (like during our recent Thanksgiving dinner, for which I paid the price). But I deal with these less

and less all the time. You, too, will reach this point. Unlike mourning the loss of a loved one, when acceptance brings its own mini-mourning due to the guilt which accompanies it, there is a certain pride in reaching this point in this mourning process for an FMer. Though we are unable to conquer the condition, we can overcome the mental, emotional, and physical effects of it. Thus, we win!

Today—2019—I find it interesting to go back and read how I felt after two years of dealing with FM. I was still dealing with it. Now, twelve years later, it's life. It's normal. It's no big deal. Yes, I still read ingredient labels. I still miss a few foods. I still need to be careful when eating out. But I'm no longer frustrated. I'm no longer angry. I'm just living my normal.

These steps may come as listed in the order given, or not; or in any combination. You may skip a step or two. Awareness will be your key to "successful mourning." What is successful mourning? Not falling into the depths of depression, not driving your friends and family away, and finding ways to accept and live with this problem while still feeling like you have a full life are some of the signs of successful mourning. In other words, learning to accept and deal with your new life is successful mourning.

Additional Information

"It is believed that up to 36% of the European population has fructose malabsorption in a more or less severe form, and approximately one-half of affected individuals are symptomatic"[5].

This figure is estimated to be far higher in the United States (Could this be related to the extensive additives in our foods, such as HFCS, which is rarely used outside the U.S?). Unfortunately, it has been a little-known condition, even among the medical community, resulting in frequent lack of proper diagnosis.

Another result of this lack of familiarity with FM is the general public, acquaintances, friends, family, and even some medical personnel may respond to the FMers diagnosis with doubt. It sounds so odd and unhealthy; people often have difficulty grasping that it is a genuine condition which deserves respect.

In a survey of 33 Oregon family physicians, internists, and nurse practitioners which I initiated while researching the first edition of this book, of the twelve who responded, only four respondents were even vaguely familiar with FM, with the same number being familiar with breath hydrogen testing (not necessarily the same ones). *None were familiar with breath hydrogen testing for FM, which must be done specifically for fructose.* Surprisingly, after doing the survey, there were two respondents who said they "may" be inclined to familiarize themselves with FM and one who said "no" to familiarization. Thankfully, the remaining respondents indicated they would definitely be familiarizing themselves with FM. My question is, why would any primary health care provider not want to familiarize themselves with FM? Hopefully, over the last twelve years, these numbers have improved.

The importance of primary care physicians being knowledgeable of FM becomes obvious when one considers that many believe irritable bowel syndrome (IBS) to be a catch-all for an unexplained group of symptoms, not a diagnosis. By definition, a syndrome is not a diagnosis but a group of recognized symptoms. The dictionary defines syndrome as

"1. group of identifying signs and symptoms, 2. things that form a pattern."

IBS is a diagnosis of exclusion. If your doctor has diagnosed IBS but has not ruled out other causes, insist on further testing. Another way some view IBS is as a general term covering all disorders of the bowel.

It is estimated as many as 45-75% of those "diagnosed" with IBS actually have FM. Others may have lactose intolerance, gluten intolerance, yeast intolerance, or more serious conditions, such as Crohn's disease, diverticulitis, or colitis. Proper testing is essential. What if I had accepted prescription laxatives without question? Many other symptoms would likely have continued.

The depression associated with FM is thought to have a connection with the folic acid associated with FM. Clinical trials have shown, of those who tested positive for FM, average folic acid levels were lower than normal.

"Folic acid deficiency may contribute to the development of mental depression"[5]. (See the chapter on depression.)

While low folic acid levels are associated with cardiovascular disease and neural-tube defects in newborns,

"folic acid supplementation was found to reduce the relative risk for the development of colon carcinoma (cancer). These findings suggest that fructose malabsorption could be a risk factor in the development of these diseases."[5]

The systemic inflammation associated with FM is also believed to have detrimental long-term effects. Joint pain, allergies, heart attack, stroke, and premature aging are a few of the possible conditions associated with inflammation.

These findings help to support my theory that anything which causes such a vast array of symptoms must have some associated long-term effects, which is dramatically opposed to the information I was given upon diagnosis–that there are no long term effects of FM. This is one more reason primary care providers should familiarize themselves with FM.

Xylose isomerase is an enzyme that purportedly converts fructose to glucose in the small intestine and may help with FM symptoms. I have not tried this enzyme.

One doctor strongly suggested I become a vegan. He said it would heal my problems. After consideration, I decided to give it six months. Bad decision. I incurred more problems than I've had in years. Vegan or vegetarian diets rely heavily on legumes and lintels. Both of which are unfriendly to the FMer. After cutting them out, I was unable to get enough protein. This was evidenced by my fingernails curling. Additionally, I experienced more symptoms than I had for several years. I did stick with the vegan diet for six months, but not a day longer. Six months after stopping the vegan diet, my nails were back to normal.

The moral of this story is, while vegan or vegetarian diets may be great for some, they don't work well for the FMer.

Dietary Changes – Going Organic

While considering the potentially destructive effects of pesticides, herbicides, dyes, and other alterations (all of this I call poisons) to our foods, we realized we had both been considering "going organic" for years, but we were both too cheap to convince ourselves to do it. Face it, organic is more expensive. After much discussion and mental financial tug-of-war, we determined it was time to switch to organic foods. Why would two professed cheapskates make a decision which could effectively double their food bill?

Consider milk. By buying organic fat-free milk, we usually pay the same for a half gallon that we used to pay for a full gallon of non-organic milk. This seems insane until you consider what has gone into that **non**-organic gallon of milk. Besides probably being a genetically altered animal, chances are, the feed the cow eats has been altered, poisoned, or contains animal bi-products. The cow has probably been shot full of hormones, antibiotics, and other medications to help it grow, produce more, and stay healthy despite not being free to exercise and being fed a diet unnatural to cows. After the cow is milked, the milk undergoes processing. Consequently, the regular (poison) milk we drink has at least a triple poisoning to it: feed, cow, milk. To me, that just does not sound healthy. Don't forget; this includes milk products like cheese, ice cream, and sour cream.

Milk exemplifies only one food. Read a few labels. Do a bit of math. Add all the artificial additives, chemicals, dyes, irradiation, hormones, antibiotics, genetically modified organisms (GMOs), etc. in all the different foods you consume, and you may be eating the equivalent of a full meal, or at least a snack, each day of nothing but poisons. Then add to this the products we put on our skin. Medication patches work so well because the skin readily absorbs what is on it. The point is, how many artificial additives can we consume before our bodies are affected by them?

With proper nutrition being a concern, the fact that

"75 published studies have found that organic food is more nutritious than nonorganic,"[12]

is just one more reason to take a closer look at organics. This means the vitamin and mineral levels of organic foods have shown to be higher than those of non-organic foods. I cannot help but think they would have to be more nutritious when they are not full of poisons.

We have found ways to reduce the financial impact of going organic. We shop at Grocery Outlet, an outlet store in the West for groceries, and they now carry a variety of organic products. Unfortunately, being an outlet store, the products come and go. We stock up when we find products we like. We watch the other stores for sales on organics; most stores now have at least a small organic section. We have also found a couple of direct sources for organics in the form of local growers. You may be able to find organic growers at your local farmers market. If you are fortunate enough to live in a city with grocers who specialize in organic and natural foods, the search for organics will be much easier for you.

Growing your own is also an option. Even apartment dwellers can plant window gardens. This is one more way we can take control of what sometimes seems an out-of-control condition.

If all-organic is budget-prohibitive, you may want to restrict organic purchases to those having the greatest impact. When buying organic, choose thin-skinned or no skin items, such as milk, eggs, celery, lettuce, zucchini, etc. Then you can buy non-organic thick-skinned items: oranges, bananas, pomegranates, nuts, etc. If you choose to do this, keep in mind that these foods can also take in poisons just like they take in water (think of the color in carnations), so this is a compromise.

According to the definition provided by the National e-Commerce Extension Initiative at http://srdc.msstate.edu/ecommerce/curricula/farm_mgmt/glo ssary.htm

"To be labeled organic, all fresh or processed foods sold in the United States, including imports, must be produced according to the national organic standards and certified by an inspection agency accredited by the USDA. Before their crops can be certified, all organic farmers must use only approved materials. They must develop an organic farm management plan, keep detailed records, and be inspected annually by an accredited certification agency. All companies that manufacture organic food products must follow similar strict requirements."

This definition agrees with those provided by other sites. The Organic Trade Association's website at http://www.ota.com/organic/faq.html provides an excellent source for information regarding organic products.

A few words on "natural." It has no meaning on anything but meat. There are no guidelines or regulations guiding or limiting its use. There are a few "natural" products we have used, but we also researched these products to discover exactly what their use of the word "natural" means. For meat, the USDA requires products to be free of artificial ingredients, colorings, preservatives, and unnecessary processing. We used to purchase a local "natural" beef. Our research showed it to be locally raised, in pastures, eating the untreated grass grown in those pastures, without being forced to consume corn (corn fed is not a good thing, cows are not designed to consume corn, and it makes them ill without the use of antibiotics), using no growth hormones, antibiotics, or other artificial enhancements. While this beef does not have the "certified organic" label, it has been grown and produced in essentially the same manner as organic beef. The grower has simply decided against the expense of certification. Additionally, it may mean the pastures on which the cow is fed have not gone an appropriate amount of time without prohibited substances to be certified, or it is too near areas which use chemicals to be certified organic.

From the FM standpoint, I never need to worry about HFCS being used in organic products. HFCS may be made from corn, but it is *not* organic. This allows me to be able to eat some snacks and packaged products I would not be able to consume in non-organic foods. Eating organic does not mean I can stop reading labels. I still need to verify the product does not contain one of the many foods I am unable to eat. But it does make it easier.

Another thing we have noticed since our switch to organics. It tastes better. For example, the milk we discussed earlier, we noticed a subtle, yet distinctly different, taste from non-organic milk. For example, it dawned on me why our milk had been so "dull"; I had picked up a half-gallon of milk at a store which did not have organic milk, meaning I had to buy the non-organic brand. Even I was surprised by the revelation. Meat is also different. If you are over the age of 50, you may remember meat having more flavor, marbling, and color. When you buy organic, it still does. Tomatoes–our families deserve a wonderful, red, juicy, flavorful fruit; not the anemic looking, woody-textured, flavorless imitator we see today.

There have been aspects to going organic which have surprised me. When I make a meal or send lunch with my husband knowing it is all-organic, there is a sense of relief, coupled with pride. By combining sound nutrition with organic food, I know I am providing my family the healthiest meals I possibly can. This is especially important to me due to the concern about the lack of variety FM has caused in our lives.

Going organic has given me back some of the control I lost when diagnosed. In addition to mourning the loss of food as I knew it, depression for me was aggravated by the loss of control. FM became the controller of my diet; food choices were no longer mine. Now, when I find a food I can eat, which seems to defy the restrictions, I have accomplished something, I have taken back some control. Organic has given me something to focus on other than what I am unable to eat. It has put a positive element of eating back into my life. It has empowered me. Organic is my version of "making lemonade out of lemons."

Additionally, shopping is not nearly as depressing when buying organic. Without the constant threat of HFCS, there are far more options open to me. Though we live in a small town, when we get to a city with one of those wonderful food stores which specialize in organic foods, it is empowering to be able to walk down every aisle of the store and know I can find things I can eat. Living in a small town, finding organics is a challenge, but I love a good challenge.

When visiting my daughter's family in Maryland during the birth of our grandson, they seemed quite unflustered by my eating restrictions. They cook from scratch anyway and use primarily organic foods.

Rather than referring to either organic or "regular" food, I refer to organic or poison foods. Perhaps doing so will help you.

If you still are not convinced that going organic may help with your FM struggles, perhaps you will respond to the "green" argument. Organic farming is much friendlier to the environment. Non-organic farming uses tremendous quantities of herbicides, pesticides, and chemical fertilizers, which are not only on and in the food we eat but also make their way into our lakes, rivers, oceans, and even the underground water. Of course, this can also affect wildlife, such as the fish and seafood we consume. Surely, if we are willing to absorb the extra costs for other green products, we will be more than willing to do so with the food we consume.

Eating Out

As much as I would like to conclude this section with one word—don't—this is not a realistic solution. The challenge of eating out with FM is one which must be mastered by each FMer in a way which best suits the individual. It is not easy. Your companions may find it embarrassing or annoying. Restaurants are problematic in that you rarely know what the ingredients are. Think about it; onions and garlic are used extensively in cooking. Though I really can't blame chefs, onions add flavor.

For the sake of your health and well-being, speak up. This applies whether deciding on a restaurant or choosing from the menu. Never be shy about explaining you are very restricted in what you can eat. I have even begun saying I have allergies rather than a restricted diet since servers often think I am "dieting" to lose weight, thus being somewhat unimportant. While FM is not technically allergies, I need them to understand the importance of my many requests. Being an honest person, this was very difficult for me, until a co-worker pointed out that it does make me sick, just not vomit sick, so I should not feel guilty. After reviewing my own list of symptoms, I agree, it does make me sick.

Though I would love to be able to say what you can order in any given restaurant, we are so limited on restaurants in our small town that I lack the experience needed to do so. What I can recommend, and probably more useful in the long run, are some general guidelines.

- Salads: Request items like onions and croutons be omitted.

- Salad dressing: Learn to enjoy salad without it, ask for a lemon wedge on the side to squeeze on the salad, stick with oil and vinegar, or have a small container of an acceptable homemade dressing of your choice in your purse or pocket.
- Meats: Request no extra sauces be added.
- Gravy: Be cautious, ask if they make it in-house, many restaurants use gravy mixes or canned, which probably contain HFCS, especially brown gravy. Wheat flour is also used to make most gravy.
- French Fries: These can lead to confusion. They should be safe to eat. However not all French fries are "real." Some are mashed potatoes with other stuff mixed in, like onion powder, which have been formed into fries.
- Try to order foods as basic as possible. Plain steak, plain veggies, baked potato, etc.
- Know the menu before going; it saves time, frustration, and the possibility of leaving without eating. Most restaurants list their menus on the internet or in the phone book. If necessary, get a copy of the menu from the restaurant before going.
- Don't be afraid to ask if an item contains HFCS, garlic, or onions. The server may need to ask the chef or read the label.
- Avoid rush hours in restaurants. This allows the server to give more individualized service and the chef time to make exceptions.

- Breakfasts are usually easier to order.
- Eggs and omelets are usually safe, though be cautious of the ingredients in the omelet. It will probably require holds/adds.
- Breakfast fried potatoes often contain onions, be sure to ask or stick with hash browns. Though it may be wise to verify they don't add onions to their hash browns and that they are fresh, not frozen. Many frozen hash browns contain unsafe ingredients.
- Avoid cured meats such as bacon since they are often cured with honey or molasses.
- Avoid processed meats such as sausage; they frequently contain or may be cured with unacceptable ingredients.
- Though some FMers have been able to eat real sourdough bread, most in restaurants will not be real. In theory, the souring process destroys the fructans. If you do try, be sure to limit the amount.
- Avoid soups; chances are, they contain onions. Ask before ordering.
- Place a roll of Smarties® (known as Rockets in Canada) or glucose tablets next to your plate, eating one occasionally to help guard against any hidden fructose. Remember, this can backfire if the food contains fructans, such as onions.

Gatherings, such as employee dinners and receptions, pose another problem. Catered foods should all be labeled "Dangerous for FMers." We have decided the best way for me to deal with these situations is to eat before going and then chose (if a buffet) the closest things to "safe" I see.

When traveling, rather than eating out the entire trip, we take a cooler filled with possibilities.

- oatmeal muffins (both savory & sweet), included in the recipe section
- sandwiches
- sandwich fixings, such as GF bread (I like to cut each slice in half making them thinner since GF bread is rather dense, it makes better sandwiches), mayo, meat, tuna salad, PB&J, etc.
- water (by the gallon, which we use to refill our glass water bottles)

You get the idea. When we run out of ingredients, we just go grocery shopping. Not only is this much safer, it's also far less expensive than eating out.

Help for the Hurting

What to do to stop the symptoms caused by FM is a big question. The most obvious answer is to stop consuming things that cause problems. This is easier said than done.

If you know or suspect you will be eating something you should not eat, take a dextrose (glucose) tablet before eating to help correct the fructose/glucose ratio. If you cannot find these, the candy, *Smarties®* (known as Rockets in Canada), may be of assistance. This sweet little candy's first ingredient is dextrose. Even better, there is no HFCS. Of course, they are not organic and contain food dyes. Also, one little roll contains a whopping 100 calories. Be aware; these will **not** help with fructans; in fact, they may exacerbate the problem with fructans. If I suspect a food item may have an unfavorable ratio, I will eat a few *Smarties®*. While eating out at a recent dinner theater, I kept a roll next to my charger (the bottom plate which remains throughout the meal), eating a few with each course. This even got me through a small glass of Merlot and the establishment's marvelous, signature grape salad. It may have added an extra 100 calories, but it made my evening far more pleasant.

Unfortunately, it seems regardless how careful the FMer is with diet, something sneaks its way in and we find ourselves in pain, full of gas, dashing to the bathroom, with bile in our throats, feeling like a balloon, battling a headache, or just feeling crappy and lethargic. Now what?

There are ways to battle the symptoms which otherwise seem to defy the typical remedies. Listed below are some things which have helped me.

Rice bag: If you are not familiar with these, you are in for a treat. They are the microwave-age version of a hot water bottle. Typically it is a cloth envelope of various shapes and sizes which is filled with rice, flax, corn, or wheat. The one I use most is filled with flax and rice. It can be heated in the microwave for warmth or left in the freezer for a cold compress. You can make it yourself or purchase one in stores, on the internet, or at craft fairs. They are quite simple to make with instructions readily available on the internet. Some also have added ingredients such as lavender or cinnamon for aromatherapy purposes. I have several of these in various sizes for different uses which I keep in the freezer and available to pop in the microwave. I even have a pair of rice bag booties for those times when I am unable to sleep because my feet are cold.

Stomach pain:

Heat.

Heated rice bag on tummy. Be careful not to overheat the rice bag; it can cause burns. But you will want it as hot as possible.

Hot shower, hot bath, or hot tub. When showering in the morning, I discovered my night-long pain would often be gone or reduced after my morning shower. When pain was especially bad, a soak in our hot tub gave me instant relief. However, if the pain included a lot of gas, as soon as I got out of the hot tub, at least some of the pain returned.

Headache:

Frozen rice bag on head.

Ibuprofen (Advil).

Drink water.

Hot shower (the steam helps open swollen sinus passages, and it's relaxing).

Migraine:

A woman I used to work with told me a trick her doctor suggested. Take eight hundred milligrams of Advil (four over the counter) and four hundred milligrams of Excedrin (two over the counter). Four hours later, take another four hundred milligrams of Advil (I have found liqui-gels work better and faster). This works well. The caffeine in the Excedrin will keep me awake all night, so I try not to do this after two o'clock. As always, check with your doctor.

Frozen rice bag on head.

Dark room.

Acid indigestion or bile in throat:

Baking soda, be sure to follow the directions on the box,

- add ½ teaspoon to 4 ounces water…

Though the above works well for an attack, for avoiding attacks, the opposite works well. By fighting reflux with baking soda or antacids, we lower the necessary acid in our stomach, thus telling our body to produce more acid. An endless cycle. Instead, daily ingestion of a small amount of apple cider vinegar helps to avoid reflux. It's also purported to help heal leaky gut.

Gas:

Heated rice bag.

Drink water.

Exercise. As uncomfortable as you may be, a walk or calisthenics can be quite helpful.

Simethecone, such as extra-strength Gas-X®.

Puffiness/Systemic Swelling:

Ibuprofen or a similar anti-inflammatory may be of some help.

I have found Benadryl (I use liqu-gels whenever possible) to be helpful and understand other FMers also have.

Constipation:

MiraLAX® (check with your doctor first). Be sure it is thoroughly dissolved before drinking.

Water.

Interesting reading material.

Since becoming extremely strict with my diet, I seldom have problems with this. So I would have to say the best thing is preventative. Avoid offending foods.

Diarrhea:

While this is not an area in which I have experience (check with your doctor), my research does show you should be very conscious of remaining hydrated. Drink plenty of water. For excessive diarrhea, you may want to try something which will replace electrolytes, such as Gatorade (if you can tolerate this), but be sure to read labels; some Gatorade contains HFCS.

The best thing, as with constipation, is preventative. Avoid offending foods.

Legal:

Because I am not an attorney, I would suggest you consult one before pursuing the following. If you have been challenged by problems on the job due to the effects of FM, it is my understanding that FM is covered by the American's with Disabilities Act (ADA). As a payroll professional, I read about a Supreme Court decision which allowed that an employee with bowel/bladder problems must be relieved from duty to attend to bodily needs regardless of break periods (unsure of the source). Also, the ADA Amendments Act of 2008, which took effect January 2009, specifies a list of *major life activities*, including major bodily functions such as bowel and bladder, as covered by the ADA. For those of you with diarrhea reactions, this could allow you to run to the much-needed bathroom, despite it not being break-time. For those of us with constipation problems, this may provide protection when we get "stuck" on the toilet and exceed our break or arrive late to work.

Depression

Due to the relationship between FM and depression, as well as the likelihood of an onset of depression after a diagnosis of FM, we feel the inclusion of a chapter about depression essential to the completeness of this book. Most of this chapter is an adaptation of two papers I wrote on the subject. As a result, it may include more information than is necessary for the scope of FM, but since many FMers may have been fighting depression for extended periods of time, we did not edit it as much as we could have.

Why is depression associated with FM? The unabsorbed fructose which has passed on to an FMers lower intestine then bonds with tryptophan, thus rendering the tryptophan unabsorbable. Tryptophan is an amino acid needed to make serotonin, which helps guard against depression. Some call it a happy neurotransmitter. Plus, tryptophan becomes melatonin, the substance that tells us to sleep when it becomes dark. Thus, FMers have problems sleeping, and a lack of sleep contributes to depression. Is it just me, or is there is a pattern forming here? On the brighter side, when we stop consuming fructose, we start producing tryptophan so the depression goes away or at least improves.

Foods high in tryptophan include shrimp, sesame seed, and milk. For a more complete listing, see the list beginning on page 110. Also available are supplements, though as always, caution should be used in this area. In 1989, an outbreak of an auto-immune illness called eosinophilia-myalgia syndrome (EMS) was attributed to L-tryptophan, resulting in the ban of this supplement in the United States. The problem was ultimately traced to one manufacturer in Japan. In 2002, the FDA removed their ban on its sale. Remember, FMers do not need to supplement, they simply need to stop consuming fructose so the tryptophan can absorb.

There are other factors which affect the absorption of tryptophan. Vitamin B6 is also necessary for the conversion of tryptophan to serotonin. Thus a deficiency in B6 may also contribute to depression. B6 is found in bananas, salmon, turkey, spinach, and hazelnuts, to name a few. Additionally, there are conditions and lifestyle choices which can reduce the conversion of tryptophan to serotonin: smoking, high sugar intake, alcohol abuse, excessive consumption of protein, hypoglycemia, and diabetes. As always, be sure to have your physician check your B6 levels and determine a dosage before beginning any supplements.

According to the National Institute of Mental Health, 9.5% of the population of the United States suffers from depression in any given year. Yet, depression remains vastly misunderstood, the butt of jokes, ridicule, and disbelief. It is referred to by some as an excuse for laziness. Although the long list of famous sufferers includes Abraham Lincoln, Samuel Clemens, Sergey Rachmaninoff, Irving Berlin, Walt Whitman, and Vincent van Gogh; acceptance of victims has been slow.

As a survivor of clinical depression, I know the embarrassment, reality, pain, and disruption of depression firsthand. During my initial bout with major depression many years ago, I had no idea what it was and feared I was going insane. By my second episode, I knew what it was and sought to educate myself further, as well as received extensive treatment. However, the embarrassment of a mental disorder limited my circle of confidants regarding my condition and treatment to three people. Years later, with maturity and good health, I determined never to keep silent regarding this subject again. If my experience or knowledge could help others, I must share it.

Depression, a mood disorder, has many degrees of severity ranging from mild "blues" of short duration to psychotic depression. The three major types of depression are bi-polar disorder, dysthymia, and major depressive disorder (also known as clinical depression).

Seasonal affective disorder (SAD), also known as winter depression, is a mild form of depression characterized by symptoms only during the winter. While SAD is almost unknown in tropical locations, it can be quite common in locations with extended winter, darkness, and rain. When coupled with another form of depression, this can result in an extreme depressive period.

Dysthymia is chronic, low-level depression. During a life crisis, the sufferer may develop major depressive disorder, not in place of, but in addition to dysthymia.

Reactive depression, also known as adjustment disorder with depressed mood, is depression brought on as the result of an occurrence, such as the death of a loved one or the loss of a job. This is a category of last resort, used only if the depression does not fit another term.

Major depressive disorder is an overwhelming depression with many symptoms. Some of these symptoms seem inconsistent with the term "depression," and will be discussed in detail later in this chapter.

Melancholic depression, according to the Diagnostic and Statistical Manual of Mental Disorders (DSM-IV) is a state of complete anhedonia, the inability to experience pleasures.

Psychotic depression is characterized by delusions and hallucinations. This is an extremely severe depression which can result from untreated depression of other forms.

Bi-polar depression (or disorder) is characterized by episodes of depression followed by episodes of manic behavior, characterized by euphoria, inflated self-esteem, and temporary loss of reality. Though a mood disorder within the depression spectrum, it is considered a separate disorder and is treated differently than depression.

Major depressive disorder affects different people differently. While one person may have trouble eating or sleeping, another may eat and sleep excessively. Fidgeting, hand wringing, and pacing may highlight one person's movements, while slowed speech, reaction time, and body movements mark another person's movements. Some people have many symptoms of depression, others have only a few. For some, it is obvious they are sufferers of depression; while for others, day-to-day functions may be relatively unimpaired.

In addition to the often mentioned overwhelming sadness, despair, hopelessness, and loss of ability to experience pleasure, there are less publicized symptoms of depression. Overreaction to minor occurrences, inability to make decisions, inability to concentrate, memory problems, anger, and unexplained aches and pains are notable in sufferers. The inability to do basic things such as: get out of bed, clean house, bathe, or fix a meal is an often misunderstood symptom of depression. This inability is not laziness or a choice; it can be as debilitating as a broken leg is to walking.

Symptoms of depression are many, varying by severity of the depressed state and individual. The symptoms may last for weeks, months, or years. The following list is not to be considered all-inclusive, nor is an individual likely to experience all of them.

Concentration Problems
Easy Loss of Temper
Difficulties Making Decisions
Social Withdrawal
No Desire for Pleasurable Activities
Lack of Appetite
Increased Appetite
Memory Problems
Excessive Sleeping
Insomnia
Restlessness
Excessive Crying
Decreased Energy
Thoughts of Death or Suicide
Increased Irritability
Difficulty Remembering
Difficulty Making Decisions
Lack of Motivation
Chronic Fatigue
Apathy
Complaining
Neglect of Personal Appearance
Persistent physical symptoms which do not respond to treatment, such as: headaches, digestive disorders, and chronic pain–could this be a result of FM?
Feelings of: sadness, emptiness, hopelessness, dysphoria, guilt, worthlessness, and pessimism

With typical depression, the patient will eat and sleep less; while atypical depression is characterized by oversleeping, overeating, and resulting rapid weight gain. This is usually the type I fight. I seldom do anything in the "typical" manner.

The diagnosis of depression should be made by a qualified professional such as a psychologist or psychiatrist. A review of all medications, including herbal remedies, over-the-counter drugs, alcohol, and illegal drugs should be included. Additionally, a medical examination is called for if there are physical symptoms present. Perhaps, with what we now know about FM, a breath hydrogen test should be standard.

Depression is highly responsive to treatment, which takes two forms, psychotherapy and medications. For mild to moderate depression, psychotherapy is considered most appropriate, while more severe cases usually require medication with therapy. Recovery rates have been shown to be significantly higher when psychotherapy and drug therapy are used in combination. Medication relieves the physical symptoms, which allows the user to concentrate on psychotherapy, which teaches coping skills.

Helping the patient gain insights into the causes of depression, psychotherapy takes two forms. Interpersonal therapy focuses on managing relationships which cause and exacerbate depression. Cognitive, also known as behavioral, therapy works to change negative thinking and behavior associated with depression. After significant improvement, therapists may use psychodynamic therapy, which focuses on resolving the patient's conflicted feelings.

It is important to remember that therapists differ in ability just as any doctor, mechanic, accountant, or teacher does. If the therapy is not beneficial or if there is poor therapist/patient rapport, a new therapist should be sought, just as one would do if their mechanic's work was ineffective.

Drug therapy is a useful and necessary form of treatment for depression and should be used in conjunction with psychotherapy. While medications allow for symptomatic relief, much like cold medications, they do not treat the disease. There are three basic forms of medications for the treatment of depression, none of which are habit forming, though stopping the medication must be done slowly to prevent reoccurrence of symptoms. Depression medications are not speed, a happy pill, or a substitute for therapy. Additionally, sedatives are not anti-depressants.

The three forms of anti-depressants are tricyclics, selective serotonin reuptake inhibitors (SSRI's), and monoamine oxidase inhibitors (MAOI's). Each type has its own uses, as well as side effects. The type of depression helps to determine which medication type will be effective.

Tricyclics are an older form of anti-depressant. Potential side effects may be: dry mouth, constipation, bladder problems, sexual problems, blurred vision, dizziness, and drowsiness in the daytime. While few users suffer all or even several of these symptoms, most usually disappear after adjusting to the medication.

Selective serotonin reuptake inhibitors (SSRI's) are one of the new medications for depression and affect neurotransmitters such as dopamine or norepinephrine. They have fewer side effects than tricyclics; headache, nausea, nervousness, insomnia, agitation, and sexual problems may plague the user.

While these same side effects apply to monoamine oxidase inhibitors (MAOI's), the other new class of medications used to treat depression, additional precautions must be taken to avoid foods and drugs with high levels of tyramine, which could result in a hypertensive crisis, leading to stroke. These foods include cheese, wine, and pickles, as well as decongestants.

All anti-depressants must be taken regularly for three to four weeks, though some as long as eight, before the full therapeutic effect occurs. Medication must then continue for at least four to nine months to prevent reoccurrence. Monitoring the discontinuation of anti-depressants is essential, due to the risk of reoccurrence when abruptly stopped.

In 2006 the FDA approved the first transdermal (skin) patch, Emsam (selegiline), an MAOI inhibitor, for treatment of major depression. Using one low dose patch per day with none of the dietary restrictions associated with MAOI's should make life easier and less restrictive for patients.

Other, more radical treatment options are also available. Though these are undoubtedly out of the scope of FM, I include them for interest and completeness.

Electroconvulsive therapy (ECT), once known as shock treatment, is used only for severe cases of depression which are not responsive to other treatments. Lower levels of shock are now administered than in previous times. Confusion and memory loss are possible side effects.

Vagus nerve stimulation (VNS), in which a pacemaker-like device is implanted which sends electric impulses to the vagus nerve requires four or more medications to have been ineffective and the patient to be at least 18 years of age. Forty percent of patients have shown 50 percent or greater improvement. Side effects include hoarseness, sore throat, and shortness of breath.

Transcranial magnetic stimulation (TMS), also known as repetitive transcranial magnetic stimulation (rTMS), was developed in 1985 and has been used in the treatment of mental illness since 1995. Electromagnets deliver short bursts of energy to stimulate nerve cells in the brain. The effect is comparable to a placebo and is used when the patient has not responded to traditional therapy.

Alternative medicines include St. John's wort, ephedra, gingko biloba, echinacea, ginseng, and zinc, though no significant evidence has shown any of these to be beneficial. Care must be used when taking alternative medicines to consult a physician for potential drug interactions. Additionally, recent research has concluded that swimming with bottlenose dolphins for a period of at least two weeks may have some beneficial effect.[9] It could be assumed the benefit of this therapy may come more from doing something unusual, relaxing, and pleasurable than actually swimming with the dolphins. Perhaps snorkeling in the Caribbean or taking the long-dreamt-of pottery class may achieve similar results.

Obviously, for the FMer suffering from depression, the primary treatment is to control the fructose intake, thus allowing tryptophan to absorb. Psychotherapy and/or the support of other FMers may be needed to deal with the drastic change in life caused by FM.

Unfortunately, some will choose to self-medicate with drugs or alcohol. These simply exacerbate the depression through increased problems of physical, financial, legal, mental, and stress difficulties. It is debated whether substance abusers have an increased rate of depression or if depression brings about substance abuse.

Though chemical imbalances in the brain are thought by many to be a cause of depression, these imbalances usually disappear upon completion of psychotherapy and this without medication. This suggests that perhaps the imbalance is a physical response to psychological distress. However, the fact that some types of depression run in families (bi-polar and major depressive disorder), suggests that there is a biological connection. This can once again be debated by those arguing that social learning and coping factors learned within the family contribute to the hereditary link.

One might wonder if the chemical imbalance is a result of other imbalances, such as those associated with FM as described at the beginning of this chapter.

Certain high blood pressure and arthritis medications can have a drug interaction which can bring about depression. Life events such as medical problems (like FM), financial difficulties, loss of loved ones, and loneliness experienced by those without proper coping skills are known triggers for depression. Elderly in institutions, diabetics, the socially isolated, and adolescents at the onset of puberty are at increased risk. People with other psychological disorders, especially anxiety disorders, have a higher rate of depression.

Commonly, those who suffer from depression share certain traits. They include pessimism, unrealistic expectations, overly self-critical, low self-esteem, perfectionism, greater dependency needs, low self-efficacy (low self-worth), and external locus of control (getting one's sense of self from sources outside self, such as loved ones, need for recognition, and surroundings). For those who possess these traits or have a family history of depression, perhaps possible preemptive measures would aid in reducing depression occurrence. Counseling before depression or even classes or self-help books on building self-esteem may be beneficial.

Many of the traits mentioned above could be used to describe me. For example, if it were not for that trait of perfectionism, the first edition of this book would have been published six months sooner. Thankfully, fewer apply today than in previous years.

After adolescence, women are twice as likely to suffer from depression as men. This holds true regardless of racial or ethnic background and is the same in eleven other countries as well. There have been many theories regarding the reasoning for this difference in rates. Among them are hormonal differences, social role differences, and cultural differences. Many women experience pre-menstrual syndrome (PMS), with the emotional symptoms very closely mimicking depression. Additionally, postpartum depression, which can, in extreme cases, lead to major depressive disorder, is thought to be due to the radical change in hormones experienced after birth. I experienced my first bout of major depressive disorder post partum. It is also interesting to note that one study has shown gender as a possible influence in FM, with women exhibiting more FM than men.[13]

Social role differences play an important part in the rate of depression differences by gender. While traditionally, men have had jobs and careers which allowed them to have defined schedules, time away from home, and fulfilling feedback, women have traditionally stayed at home. The homemaker's job, while important, can often be thankless, scheduleless or routine, and confining. All of these things can contribute to depression. Even today, when many women have satisfying careers outside the home, many still retain responsibility for housekeeping, child care, and meals, which can lead to feelings of being overwhelmed, a trigger for depression.

The rate difference between genders may be due to men being less likely to seek help. Additionally, men tend to self-medicate with alcohol or drugs more often, therefore the depression may simply be masked by substance abuse. This argument can be substantiated by looking at the Amish, where alcohol use is forbidden; in whom the depression rate for men and women is equal. Of course, culture differences can be closely associated with social differences. Additionally, with culture there is the question of reliability within the reported rates. It could be that in some cultures depression is simply under-reported due to cultural norms, allowances, and expectations.

This higher incidence of depression in women begins in adolescence. Until then, boys show an equal or even higher rate than girls. This leads us to realize other possible reasons for the higher rate in women are: hormonal, reproductive, genetic/biological factors, abuse and oppression, psychological and personality characteristics, different coping mechanisms, and social expectations. The reasons are unclear.

Victims' studies have shown an increased rate of depression among women who were: molested as children, raped as an adult, physically abused, mentally abused, or sexually harassed or abused. This may be due to these actions fostering low self esteem, feelings of helplessness, self-blame, and social isolation.

Seniors citizens also show a higher rate of depress..
in women than men. Attributing to this may be the reality
that women statistically live longer, thus outliving their
spouses and suffering the loss of a loved one. This may also
explain why unmarried or widowed seniors show a higher
rate of depression. Other factors contributing to depression in
senior citizens are: forced retirement, health problems,
disability, age restrictions, caretaking responsibilities, lack of
mobility, loss of driving privileges, and social isolation.

Children also suffer from depression. Faking illness,
refusing to go to school, clinging to a parent, and worrying a
parent may die, are indicators of depression in young
children. For older children, sulking, negativity, feelings of
being misunderstood, and grouchiness may be indicatory of
depression. These symptoms make it difficult to diagnose
depression in teens, since they are also associated with teen
rebellion or emotional reactions to hormonal changes.
However, they should not be overlooked since four out of
one hundred teens are diagnosed as seriously depressed each
year.

Whether income level plays a part is also subject to
debate. Perhaps this income level factor has to do with the
ability to get treatment, though studies have shown lower
income sufferers are less likely to respond to treatment. Of
course, higher incomes may allow people to participate in a
greater variety of activities more often.

For those who have recovered from a bout with
depression, the risk of recurrence increases with each
successive depression. There are, however, steps one can
take to increase feelings of self-worth and self-respect, which
will aid in decreasing the risk of recurrence. I have survived
two major bouts with depression and have adjusted my

nd habits to include these recommendations, a few
I have discovered myself and not seen listed in any
rces.

Ways to Battle Depression:
- Set a regular schedule, including a specific time for going to bed and getting up.
- Have a morning routine which includes dressing, shoes, hair, make-up or shaving.
- Maintain clean, orderly surroundings.
- Prioritize your life.
- Limit your responsibilities, feelings of being overwhelmed are a trigger.
- Maintain financial balance. Overwhelming debt is a loss of control.
- Keep goals attainable.
- Be social, especially when feelings say not to.
- Break large tasks into small ones which are not as overwhelming.
- Get plenty of regular exercise.
- Do not accept negative thinking.
- Keep active in hobbies and other enjoyable activities.
- Do not make major life decisions without consulting others when depressed.
- Set limits, such as not eating in front of the television.
- See a professional if needed.
- For the FMer, taking control of your diet, as I have with organics, helps to achieve a feeling of control over food.

- Peer support can be invaluable in aiding self-acceptance and reducing the stigma attached to depression and seeking help. Sharing personal knowledge and coping strategies with others can help everyone involved, as well as providing social support. By seeking peer support, one can obtain a feeling of greater control, which aids greatly in repressing depression. The fact that the support is coming from peers rather than being paternalistic (such as me sharing my experiences with my child) or hierarchical (such as in a patient/councilor situation) also contributes to success. Ultimately, the better one can feel about self and surroundings, the better they will do.

To help a depressed person:
- Be encouraging.
- Make the appointment for treatment, if necessary. You may also need to take the depressed person to the appointment.
- Assure that medications are being taken.
- Provide emotional support in the form of being understanding, patient, and affectionate.
- Listen to the sufferer.
- Do not disparage their thoughts and feelings, though gently pointing out realities and hopes can be of help.
- Invite them out; depressed people isolate themselves, so be insistent, yet respectful.
- Encourage activities; take a class with them.
- Encourage exercise; do it with them.

- Never accuse someone of faking depression, laziness, or not desiring to get better.
- Always report any talk of suicide.

Suicide is the third leading cause of death in the 15 to 24 age group. It must be taken seriously. Additionally, it is the eighth leading cause of death for men, and eleventh for people of all ages. Women attempt suicide three times as often as men. The key word there is "attempt," men succeed more often.

Why is the rate of suicide increasing? Many things may attribute to this increase: it is in the spotlight, creating more diagnosis; increased substance abuse; rising stress levels due to the changing job market and unemployment; an unhealthy focus on self; television, with its accompanying exposure to violence; lack of exercise; unrealistic lifestyles and images; reduced social interaction; social media; and a lack of commitment to a greater good.

Early screening and intervention help prevent major depression with its potential for long term disability. Improving the ability of the primary care physician (PCP) to recognize depression, even mild cases, would aid in this effort. Additionally, PCP's increased understanding of the need to treat the disease through psychotherapy, rather than just the symptoms with medications, will aid in reducing depression rates.

As an FMer, if you seek help for depression, be sure your physician or therapist is aware of the FM and its accompanying tryptophan absorbency problems. You may wish to show him/her the first few pages of this chapter.

Reduced depression rates would also save expense in the form of reduced costs for employers though less absenteeism, turnover, and increased motivation as well as productivity. Nearly 19 million Americans suffer from depression resulting in direct and indirect costs of over $80 billion per year. As one of the leading causes of disability worldwide, depression demands research and respect as a disease.

Knowledge is power. Possessing this information may assist the FMer in battling this potentially disabling side effect of FM. Be aware of the symptoms. Take steps to minimize the grip or possibility of depression. Don't let FM or its partner, depression, win.

Bob's Point of View

From the First Edition:

My wife Debra was diagnosed in 2007 with FM. The good news, we finally knew why she was always hurting. The bad news, life was about to become a little more complicated.

After searching the internet and printing food lists and any other information we could find, we realized that no two lists were the same. They were, in fact, quite contradictory. I then made a list of my own, including only foods which were okay on all the different lists. The resulting list was very small. As I sat and looked at it, I wondered what we would eat. *What kind of recipes could I make with that little list?* I wanted to cook a few things Deb could eat and see if she would start feeling better. There were only five veggies on the list, and one of them she didn't like.

I mean, come on, no canned corn, corn on the cob, corn tortillas, no tomatoes, tomato sauce, tomato paste, ketchup…no onions, garlic, carrots, peas. There goes Mexican, Italian, Chinese, stew, and my favorite, the hamburger corn casserole my mom made. I hate to talk about the negatives here, but that forbidden list was huge. I went through several cookbooks trying to alter some recipes without much luck. At least I had meat, potatoes, eggs, and dairy, which helped a little.

As the weeks passed, Debra became more and more frustrated. Breakfast was easy, but making lunch for herself, dinner for us, or shopping for tolerable foods was starting to get the best of her. I cooked when I could to take some of the burden off of her, but more than once, when I made the mistake of asking what she might want for dinner, she broke down in tears. This new lifestyle was overwhelming, and she was tired of dealing with it. Shopping with her on weekends seemed to help. Reading labels while working our way down each aisle showed the difficulty of finding anything without HFCS or other forbidden additives.

Keeping morale up was not easy, but I always tried to find the bright side somewhere. Then I began to get irritated myself. We did not have any good food around the house anymore, and I could not even find a quick snack. Just as couples say "we're" pregnant, "we" have FM. Yes, Debra, the kids, and I were all in the same boat. Deb was the only one feeling the real pain, but we were all feeling the hunger.

As if the problems we were working through at home due to FM were not bad enough, try going to someone else's house for dinner. At first, they would cook as they normally did. Deb would pick through trying to find something she could eat, not wanting to make a big deal of it. Then the questions would arise. "Can't you eat that?" "No." "Well, what can you eat?" Deb would then try to explain what she could not eat until I would interrupt and suggest she stick with what she could eat, it would not take as long. After explaining this, most people would just stare with a puzzled look on their faces. While the majority are still baffled, they will at least attempt to make a plan with Deb before cooking.

When we were first married, we learned that eating out, wine tasting, and trying different types of food was fun. We went to all the places in town (small town) and tried different things on the menu. This also gave us a good excuse to take a road trip by ourselves or with friends and family. Whenever we went on vacation, eating new and different food was beginning to take over as the best part of the trip.

This seems funny to me now, but when we first started going out after Deb was diagnosed with FM, no one was laughing. What was once a quiet, relaxing, romantic, fun night became a stressful, complicated evening without much romance or fun. We simply quit going out to dinner for a while. It just was not worth the money for the added stress it would bring.

Breakfast was still good. Thank goodness for breakfast! We could eat out while enjoying the restaurant and the atmosphere with few problems. Despite not being able to have syrup or jelly on her pancakes (before discovering fructans/wheat is problematic) and steering clear of cured ham and sausage, breakfast was still a good time.

Lunch was a pain, but is cheaper than dinner, so we still went out occasionally. We would pick up our menus and study them, trying to discern something safe for Deb to eat. Usually, before we had decided, an unsuspecting waitress would approach the table. "Run!" I thought, "You don't know what you're getting yourself into." No, this was not going to be an easy tip, with Deb asking if the gravy was made in house or came in a package. Does it have HFCS in it? MSG? Corn flour? Does the meat have a rub, brine, or a sauce on it? What are the veggies, and can I substitute? By this time, the confused looking server would usually force a smile and offer to ask the cook. Usually, she would return with "the cook's not sure," and offer an uneducated guess of her own.

By this time I would be a bit embarrassed. I understood Deb wanted to order something which would not make her spend the rest of the day in misery, but I'm just not the type to run the wait staff around in circles trying to accommodate me. If the food is not the best or the service is not good, rather than saying anything, I may not tip as well or simply not return, but normally, I am not one to complain.

Hopefully, by now we would find something easy, very basic, or (sigh) Deb might go on to the next choice on the menu and go through it all again. Yes, by this time I was irritated. We may have ended up having wonderful food, wine, or a good beer for me, but my patience and understanding were shot.

We had a few bad lunch experiences, but in the mean time, we were learning. We were both new at this FM thing. We didn't know how to deal with it. We were in denial. We did not want to accept this new life. But we did learn patience. We gained experience and learned to have a good time. I guess you could say lunch was our practice, how we learned we could go out to dinner again and enjoy ourselves.

Admittedly, I miss the old days, when we could go out and eat or drink whatever we wanted to, but we've learned so much about food, additives, and preservatives, I am sure we eat healthier now. Though Deb still experiences pain, from unknowingly eating something bad or from just being defiant and eating a brownie, I encourage her that if she will eat cautiously for a few days in a row and get her system cleaned out, we can try something new in her diet. We keep trying to add new foods to the okay list, or at least to the tolerable list.

The doctor says there are no long-term effects, but with the headaches, depression, bloating, and other symptoms we have associated with the way she eats, I think there is more to it than the doctors know at this time.

97

So what can I tell you, the reader? It will take time and patience. During that time, get on the internet and search for information which is increasing continually. Take control of your life, eat right, and exercise. This will all help with the associated depression. If someone you live with has FM, encourage them to eat foods they can easily tolerate for a few days then pick one of their favorite foods to try. If that food causes discomfort, depending on the severity, it may be able to be eaten in smaller quantities. Experimentation is the only way you can increase the size of the okay list. The best way to help you through this time is to help the FMer. There is a lot of good food out there, so look at it as a challenge. Life is still good!

Twelve Years Later

It's been twelve years since we started this journey. Life is still good and getting better all the time.

When we started, our biggest problem was the lack of information. Today we are gifted with plenty of information, but there are no 100% safe guidelines. Many people have other intolerances as well as FM. It's still trial, error, elimination diets, and simple cooking with raw, unprocessed foods.

It's easier at home now. The kids are all grown and gone, which makes trying new diets easier. We've tried several over the years. They weren't all fun, but they gave us a better understanding of which foods are okay to eat.

Restaurants are easier now also. We've learned how to order, where to go, and where not to go. There's no guarantee when traveling and eating at new restaurants, but we stick to simple, easy to alter ingredients. For instance, we both enjoy a good burger. Some places offer gluten-free buns. If not, Deb will bring her own or have it lettuce wrapped.

Deb's pain used to be daily and severe. She can now go months without pain if she's good. What used to be inevitable daily pain is now more of a choice. Is it worth feeling bad to eat that piece of chocolate cake? Is her bucket close to full? If so, that questionable item is probably not the best choice. However, if she's been eating well and sees a gluten-free cake at the store or farmer's market, she can chance it. Now that she's more educated and experienced, it's her decision. She knows beforehand what kind of pain and FM hangover she's risking. Choice is freedom. Uneducated random food choices can be a disaster.

My doctor has recently suggested some specific food guidelines for me, which get thrown into the mix with FM restrictions, but it all boils down to simple, unprocessed food.

You're not going to learn this overnight, but with all the new information available now, you'll get there much faster than we did.

Remember, life is still good!

My Story – Part Two

At the time of my diagnosis, my husband, Bob, and I had recently begun enjoying trying different wines and cheeses. After my diagnosis, that stopped. Wine is not my friend, especially the sweet wines I enjoy. I can, however, have very small amounts of very dry white wine, though since I do not enjoy it, we mostly limit its use to cooking.

We also enjoyed trying new foods at new restaurants. Since restaurants are now a dangerous source of frustration, this is no longer fun. I use the term dangerous because we never know for sure what is in the food. Also, the onions I had spent forty years learning to like, only to learn they are my enemy, are used universally in restaurants.

To say the depression which has been my nemesis for years has been defeated is premature. Unfortunately, the changes FM make, coupled with the frustration of the never-ending task of figuring out what to eat, exacerbated my depression. As I have learned more and feel more control over my food choices, I have continually improved in this area.

When I was first diagnosed, I would walk into the kitchen for meal preparation, realize I had no idea what I could eat or that I was wary of the few foods I knew were okay, and then walk out. I simply could not make a meal. Not eating was easier than trying to figure out what I could eat. Thankfully, Bob is better in the kitchen than I am anyway, so he took over completely. It took three months for me to attempt dinner. Time and confidence have given us the knowledge to prepare meals with little or no frustration. Dinner can, once again, be a delight.

The grocery store was another source of total despair. It was six months before I could shop by myself. What does one buy when their favorite section had previously been produce? This, coupled with HFCS listed on so many labels, and I was lost. Try buying a loaf of bread without HFCS next time you go to the store. (More are now available, but gluten-free is limited and expensive.)

Unlike a weight-loss diet, cheating is no fun. Beyond the pain involved, I have noticed I get an FM "hangover." Systemic bloating is the most annoying price I pay. It is no fun feeling like a balloon. Add to this a headache, gas, lethargy, lack of sleep, and pain, well, cheating is not worth it.

Extended family and friends are also affected by FM. They are afraid to make me sick. They are even more perplexed about what I can and cannot eat than I was. My mom said one evening upon our arrival at her house, "I was going to have something ready to eat, but I just don't know what you can eat." As my daughters both have said, "Give me a list!" We can help alleviate some of the fear and frustration experienced by our friends and families by making and distributing lists of edibles and inedibles. Be sure to send periodic updates as your list grows. Some FMers carry a laminated list of foods to avoid when eating out to send to the chef. Remaining cheerful and not whining can help others to know it is still okay for them to enjoy food and treats, regardless of how we eat.

Then there are those people, usually casual acquaintances or strangers, who react with disbelief when told about FM. It seems when people hear of a condition with which they are unfamiliar, from someone other than a physician, some disregard it as a fad or something made-up. I realize their opinion does not matter and will probably soon be changed as this condition becomes more well known.

I would love to say I have weathered all this very well, taken it in stride, so to speak, but I cannot. When first diagnosed, I was a mess. Many tears were shed. Early on, a television commercial which showed a juicy red apple reduced me to a sobbing mess. Forget the effect the actual produce department produced. The lack of reliable information made matters much worse than they should have been.

12 Years Later

At the time of publication of the first edition of this book, more than two years after diagnosis, I was doing much better. Physically and mentally, I was in a much better place. Usually, I viewed eating restrictions as a challenge. Attitude, as in most things, is the majority of the battle. When I survived a difficult situation without getting depressed, angry, or caving in, I was proud of myself. When I gave in and ended up sick, it was a learning experience. I had no one to blame but myself. Often, I was the one who chose to eat whatever it was that made me sick. This helped me to think twice before eating the forbidden fruit (or brownie).

Now, twelve years after my diagnosis, it's no big deal. Thankfully, there is much more information available, such as the FODMAP diet. Narrowing my list of can and can't eat foods, learning of my food bucket, and adjusting/learning to cook for my needs allowed us to relax.

Learning that my strongest reactions come from fructans helped immensely. Besides becoming fructan free, I've also discovered I can have very small amounts of foods in which fructose is the problem. I even eat small apples occasionally.

Mentally, I'm in a far different place. It's no big deal. It just is. Do I still miss certain foods? Occasionally. But feeling good and healthy makes it worth it. Do I still have a tough time when eating out? While it can sometimes be a challenge to choose from the menu, I can usually find something, though I may have to ask for adjustments. One nice thing, more restaurants are including gluten-free bread as an option. Like I said before, it's no big deal. It just is.

If you have recently been diagnosed as an FMer, you may very well reach this point sooner than I did due to three reasons.

First, there is more information available to help now. Upon diagnosis, my internet research revealed very little information or research. Just one year later, when researching the paper which was the basis for the first edition of this book, there was, comparatively, a great deal of information. Now, there is far more information available. Better yet, the information is more accurate. Of course, there is still much less than we would like to find.

Also, my sincerest hope is for this book to encourage you in your acceptance and adjustment, as well as providing a resource for you, your family, and friends to understand your new life.

Lastly, I was diagnosed about six weeks after my dad's death, about the same time the trauma of his death began to subside and reality hit. This resulted in two major losses and depression hitting on two fronts.

Ultimately, it was not just the restrictions which made my early life with FM so difficult, it was taking care, only to find myself in pain, bloated, and having no idea what

I did wrong. Usually, it was those dastardly hidden onions I spent so many years learning to love which brought me to tears.

Appendix

Other Excellent Resources

The Complete Low-FODMAP Diet:
A Revolutionary Plan for Managing IBS and Other
Digestive Disorders
By: Dr. Sue Shepherd and Dr. Peter Gibson

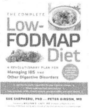

Written by members of the Monash University research
team, this is an excellent resource.

Digestive Health with REAL Food
2nd Edition
By: Aglaee Jacob, MS, RD

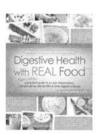

This is an interesting, easy to read book which
explains the science of fructose malabsorption and gut issues
in an easy to understand manner for those of us who don't
enjoy science. She also comes from a place of experience as
an FMer herself. Her diet recommendations are a bit

different than FODMAP, but I have tried her plan and it does work.

The Autoimmune Solution: Prevent and Reverse the Full Spectrum of Inflammatory Symptoms and Diseases
By: Amy Myers, M.D.

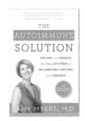

Note: she does not remove onions and garlic from the diet. If you react to fructans, this is an essential item to delete. Otherwise this is an excellent resource.

Vitamin D List

Remember, when using this or any list in this book, individual tolerances vary. The list below is only a starting point. Feel free to copy this list for your own use.

Foods High in Vitamin D
USDS Recommended Daily Amount = 400IU

Food	IU*
Beef Kidneys	32
Beef Liver	16
Butter	56
Caviar	232
Cheese	
Cheddar	12
Parmesan	28
Swiss	44
Clams	4
Cream - heavy whipping	52
Egg	35
Egg Yoke	107
Milk	
Evaporated, canned	80
Whole	40
2%	43
1%	52
Non-fat	41
Goat	12
Human	4
Mushrooms - white	181
Mushrooms - canned	21
Mushrooms - cooked	21

Soymilk		49
Fish		
	Catfish	500
	Cod	44
	Flounder	60
	Halibut	600
	Herring	1628
	Mackerel	360
	Sole	60
Oysters		320
Shrimp		152

Tryptophan List

Remember, when using this or any list in this book, individual tolerances vary. The list below is only a starting point. Feel free to copy this list for your own use.

Foods High in Tryptophan

Bananas
Chicken
Cod
Halibut
Lamb
Milk
Mustard Greens
Salmon
Sesame Seed
Shrimp
Snapper
Soybeans
Spinach
Tuna
Turkey

Recipes

This is the chapter for which you have been waiting. Or perhaps you've done what we would, perused the table of contents, then skipped right to the meat and potatoes, otherwise known as recipes.

For more recipes, look for our book, Fructose Malabsorption, the Cooking Guide. (coming soon)

Burger Gravy

1 Pound Ground Meat
Flour, we use rice or gluten free all purpose
Milk, we use flax
Salt
Pepper

Brown the meat in a skillet on medium high heat. Add flour until it stays white and will not absorb anymore. Due to the difference in amounts of fat in ground meat it is difficult to give an amount. Add about two cups of milk. If the gravy begins to thicken too much, add more milk. Simmer at a slight boil for a few minutes then reduce to low or medium low. The longer you heat (up to an hour), the better the flavor. Salt and pepper to taste.

Spoon over either mashed or baked (cut in pieces) potatoes or GF noodles or GF bread.

I usually use baked potatoes because they are quick and easy in the microwave. This is a very easy dish to throw together.

Camp Breakfast

4-5 Medium Potatoes
½ pound Ground Meat, cooked
6 slices uncured bacon, cooked and cut or crumbled
4 Eggs
1-2 Cups Cheese, cheddar, Swiss, & Jack work well
1 Cup Veggies of Choice, sliced or cubed
½ cup chopped bell peppers
Salt
Pepper

Fry potatoes, adding vegetables and cooked meat just before done. Turn the heat down to low. Add the eggs and fold in about three times only. Top with cheese and cover. When cheese has melted, remove from burner and serve.

If you stir your eggs in too long the dish will become dry. The eggs will cook as the cheese melts.

Good topped with sour cream and for other family members, salsa.

Works well wrapped in a GF tortilla as a breakfast burrito.

Nice meal for cleaning out your refrigerator.

Crab Quiche

1 Tablespoon Butter
1 Cup Shredded Crab Meat or Krab Meat
1 Tablespoon Acceptable Flour, rice or GF all purpose
1 ½ Cups Coarsely Shredded Swiss Cheese, Divided
2 Tablespoons Green Onions, green part (optional)*
9 Inch GF Pie Shell, Partially Baked
        (Can also use shredded potatoes, pressed thin like a
crust and partially baked)
3 Eggs
1 cup milk, I use flax milk
½ teaspoon salt
Dash of White Pepper or Hot-Pepper Sauce
Dash of Nutmeg

Sauté the green onions (if using) in the butter, add crab meat
and flour. Set aside. Sprinkle half the cheese in the pie shell,
then spread with the crab mixture. Sprinkle with the
remaining cheese. Whisk the eggs, cream, salt, pepper, and
nutmeg (if using) until mixed and somewhat frothy. Pour
into the pie shell and bake in pre-heated 350° oven 30-40
minutes until set and lightly browned. A knife inserted
should come out mostly clean.
I like to add broccoli heads and canned mushrooms.

Creamed Eggs
Good for breakfast or for dinner.

6 Eggs, boiled
2 Tablespoons Flour (rice flour or GF all purpose)
2 Tablespoons Butter
3 Cups Milk, more or less (I use flax milk)
Salt
Pepper

Chop the boiled eggs. I prefer the whites to be in strips.
Make rue by melting the butter in a sauce pan then adding
the flour. Add the milk. As this begins to thicken, add the
chopped eggs, whites and yolks. Salt and pepper to taste.
Dish should be thickened, but somewhat pourable.

Serve over baked or boiled potatoes. This can also be served
over GF toast.

Juice Jellies

1 Envelope Unflavored Gelatin
8 Ounces Juice
     (Be sure it is sweetened only with acceptable sugar)

In a small saucepan sprinkle the gelatin over the juice. Let stand one minute. Stir over low heat until the gelatin is dissolved, about 3 minutes. Pour into a small dish and chill until firm. Cut into squares or shapes for finger eating.

While this recipe uses juice, by serving only one juice jelly the amount of juice should not be problematic. Nice treat for children.

Fish Sauce

Mayo
Mustard or Ketchup(be careful of ingredients)
Worcestershire Sauce

Mix the ingredients together. Adjust by adding a bit more if needed.

Lettuce Wraps

Turn any sandwich into a lettuce wrap

Lettuce
Homemade Mayo
Turkey Pieces (or preferred meat)
Grated Cheese

Spread mayo on a lettuce leaf. Place turkey pieces, cheese, and mushrooms in a row on the leaf. Then roll the leaf burrito fashion.

If you prefer your roll warm, pre-warm the meat, but take care not to overheat it.

Mayo – Basic

1 Egg
1 Cup Oil
¼ teaspoon salt
2 Tablespoons White Vinegar or Lemon Juice
Dash of Pepper or Red Pepper (optional)

Add the egg, salt, vinegar, and pepper to a blender. Blend on High, adding oil one drop at a time at first, slowly increasing as mixture thickens. Stop the blender and wipe the sides, blend again. Refrigerate.

Options

Try adding 1 teaspoon of dry mustard or 1/8 teaspoon of prepared mustard (be careful of the ingredients).

Try adding ¼ teaspoon of Worcestershire sauce.

Add a bit of parsley, basil, or other flavoring.

Meatloaf

3 Pound Ground Meat-we use three different meats, such as
beef, turkey, bison (I really like it with bear)
3 Slices GF Bread, shredded
1 Cup Milk (I use flax milk)
3 Eggs
2 cups rice cereal (like rice krispies) or GF oatmeal
1 cup Celery, diced or chopped
1 Can Mushrooms, chopped
2 teaspoons Salt
2 teaspoons oregano
½ teaspoon Pepper
½ pound Uncured Bacon, diced, uncooked

Mix all ingredients together. Turn into two loaf pans.
Bake at 350° until meat thermometer reaches 180°, about 2
hours.

Carefully remove from loaf pans immediately. This will
prevent the meatloaf from absorbing all the grease it's sitting
in when you remove it from the oven.

Allow to rest 5 minutes before cutting.
Serve with acceptable ketchup or banana ketchup.

Oatmeal Muffins

Makes 12

2 cups old fashioned oats (gluten-free)

1 teaspoon cinnamon

¼ teaspoon salt

1 teaspoon baking powder

2 tablespoons chia seeds (optional)

1/4 of your favorite seed or chopped nut (I like sunflower seeds and walnuts)

1/3 fruit pieces (cherry, blueberry, strawberry all work well)

1 large egg

2 tablespoons nut butter

3/4 cup milk (any kind)

Preheat the oven to 350°F.

Grease muffin cups very well with coconut oil, line with paper liners, or use silicone muffin cups.

Mix all the ingredients together. This is easier if you have a mixer that can handle it.

Divide the mixture among the muffin cups.

Bake for 25 to 30 minutes until slightly risen and dry on top.

Remove from muffin tins onto a cooling rack to cool completely.

Muffins can be kept an airtight container on the counter for up to 5 days. Place muffins you won't eat within a few days in a ziplock or container and freeze.

To defrost: leave overnight at room temperature or microwave

For savory oatmeal muffins: omit the cinnamon and dried fruit. Stir in up to 1 cup total of ingredients like grated cheese, roasted vegetables, sautéed mushrooms. Add flavorings such as dried herbs and spices.

For other sweet oatmeal ideas: push fresh or frozen fruit (berries or cubed larger fruits are best) into each oatmeal muffin before baking.

Omelet – Basic

2 Eggs
2 Tablespoons Water
¼ teaspoon Salt
Dash of Pepper or Tabasco
½ Tablespoon Butter

Topping Possibilities:
Cheese
Uncured Bacon
Spinach
Bean Sprouts
Broccoli
Use your imagination

Heat the butter in an 8 or 10 in non-stick skillet.
Place first four ingredients in a bowl and whisk until it
begins to be frothy.
Pour the egg mixture into the medium-hot skillet. Keep
pushing the sides of the egg toward the center until the runny
egg stops flowing out to the edge. Turn down to medium-
low. Add the cheese (if using) on the whole egg, followed by
any other topping on one side of the egg only. When the egg
top is slightly moist, fold the omelet in half. Cook a bit
longer. Flip or slide onto a plate. The omelet is best if allow
to sit for a few minutes before serving.
Omelets are good topped with hollandaise sauce.

Peanut Butter Logs

1 Tablespoon Cane Sugar or Dextrose
2 Tablespoons Peanut Butter
2-3 Tablespoons Dry Milk (rice or coconut)
Chopped Nuts (optional)

Blend the sugar and peanut butter in a bowl with a wooden spoon. Add the dry milk. Make a dry still paste. Shape the paste into balls or roll into one long log to cut into one inch bite size logs. Roll in nuts, if using. Wrap. Chill in the refrigerator.

Pork Noodle Stir-Fry

9 Ounces thin rice noodles noodles
4 Tablespoons Olive Oil
1 ½ Pound Pork, cut into julienne strips
1 Cup Bean Sprouts
¼ Cup Shredded Fresh Basil
3 Tablespoons Pine Nuts, toasted
        Careful, they burn easily
2 Tablespoons Balsamic Vinegar (shouldn't be enough to
cause problem per serving (or use Worcestershire Sauce)
Sea Salt to Taste
Ground Pepper to Taste

Cook the noodles in a large saucepan of boiling water until
done. Drain, then toss with 2 tablespoons of olive oil.

Coat ta hot wok with 2 tablespoons of olive oil. Add the
Pork, cooking for 2-3 minutes. Add the bean sprouts, then
stir-fry for a minute.

Add basil, pine nuts, and balsamic vinegar. Mix well, then
add the noodles, salt, and pepper and toss.

Rice or Quinoa

1 Cup Rice or Quinoa
2 Cups Water

Add ingredients to saucepan. Cover. Bring to boil over high heat. As soon as it begins to boil, turn off heat. Let sit for 20 minutes. Do not remove lid at any time during cooking/sitting.

This is also good with broth instead of water.

Spead

1 Small Can Chopped Green Chilies
½ Cup Mayo
½ Cup Cream Cheese
½ Cup Grated Cheese

Mix ingredients well. Spread on GF bread or crackers and broil until lightly browned on top.

This works well for pizza sauce if you leave out the grated cheese.

Also works as a dip.

FODMAP Food List

Food/Drink	Sub-category/note		Fructose	Polyols	Fructans	Lactose	GOS
Acai powder		Yes					
Agar Agar		Yes					
Agave	1 teaspoon or less may be okay	No	*		*		
Ackee (AKA achee)	tinned in brine	Yes					
Alcohol-if yes, limit intake to one drink							
	Gin	Yes					
	Rum	No	*				
	Vodka	Yes					
	Tequila-despite being made from agave, I seem to tolerate small amounts						*
	Wine-dry	Yes					
	Wine-dessert	No	*				
	Whiskey	Yes					
Alfalfa Sprouts		Yes	*				
Almond Meal		No					*
Amaranth		No			*		*
Apples		No	*	*			
Apricots		No		*	*		
Artichoke							
	canned hearts	yes					
	Globe	No			*		
	Jerusalem	No	*		*		
	Pickled in oil	No	*		*		
Arugula		Yes					
Asparagus		No	*		*		
Avocado		No		*			

128

Food	Detail	Status						
Bacon	Not processed with honey or molassas	Yes						
Bamboo Shoots		Yes						
Banana			*		*			
	dried chips (check ingredients)	Yes						
	Unripe	Yes						
	Ripe	No	*		*			
Barley, Pearl		No			*		*	
Barley, Pearl, Sprouted		Yes						
Bean Sprouts	good sub for onions	Yes						
Beans - Legumes	All Dried	No			*		*	
Beans								
	Butter	No					*	
	Green	Yes						
	Fava	No	*					
	Yardlong	Yes						
Beef		Yes						
Beer		Yes						
Beet								
	root	No			*		*	
	pickled or canned	Yes						
Bell Pepper								
	green	Caution		*				
	red	Yes						
Berries								
	Blackberry	No		*				
	Blueberry	No			*			
	Boysenbery	Caution	*					
	Goji Berries	No			*			
	Raspberry	No			*			
Bitter Melon		No		*			*	
Bok Choy		Yes						
Breadfruit		Yes						

Food	Type	Status					
Broccoli							
	Chinese	Yes					
	heads only	Yes					
	stalks only	No	*				
	whole	Yes					
Broccolini		No	*				
Brussel Sprouts		No			*		
Buckwheat							
	Flakes	Yes					
	Flour	Yes					
	Groats	Yes					
	Kernels	Caution			*		
Bulgur		No			*		*
Butter		Yes					
Buttermilk		No				*	
Butternut Squash		No		*	*		*
Cabbage	can be gassy						
	Chinese	yes					
	Green	yes					
	Red	Yes					
	Savoy	No			*		
Callaloo	canned	Yes					
Cantaloupe		Caution			*		
Carob		No			*		
Carrots		Yes					
Cassava		Yes					
Cauliflower		No		*			
Celery		Caution		*			
Cereal	Read Ingredients						
	Crispix	Yes			*		
	Cornflakes	Yes					
	Rice Crisps	Yes					
Chayote		Yes					

Item	Detail	Status					
Cheese	hard cheeses	Yes		*			
Cherries, sweet		No	*				
Chewing Gum	Glee is sweetened with sugar so should be okay	No		*			
Chia Seeds		Yes					
Chicken		Yes					
Chickpeas-canned							
	canned	Caution					*
	Sprouted	No					*
Chicory Leaves		Yes					
Chilli							
	Chipotle, dried	No	*				
	Green	Yes					
	Habanero	Yes					
	Red	Yes					
Chives		Yes					
Chocolate	the only chocolate I can tolerate is white, which contains no actual chocolate						
	dark-very small amount 85%	Yes					
	milk	caution			*	*	
	white	Caution				*	
Choy Sum		Yes					
Clementine		Yes					
Coconut							
	fresh	Caution		*			
	dried	Yes					
Coconut Water		No		*	*		
Coffee		Yes					
Collard Greens		Yes					
Corn		No					
	canned baby corn	Yes					
	canned	No		*			
	creamed	Yes					
	Flour	Yes					

131

	meal	Yes					
	sweet	No		*			
	starch	Yes					
Corn Tortillas	Read Ingredients				*		
Cornmeal		yes					
Cornstarch		yes					
Cottage Cheese		Yes					
Cous Cous	gluten-free, made from maize flour	Yes					
Cranberries		No			*		
Cucumbers		Yes					
Cumquats		Yes					
Currents		No			*		
Custard Apple		No					*
Daikon		Yes					
Dates		No			*		
Dragon Fruit		Yes					
Dulse Flakes		Yes					
Durian		Yes					
Edamame		Yes					
Egg Replacer	check ingredients	Yes					
Eggplant		Yes					
Eggs		Yes					
Endive		Yes					
Feijoa		No	*		*		
Fennel							
	bulb	No		*	*		
	leaves	Yes					
Figs							
	dried	No			*		
	fresh	No	*				
Fish		Yes					
Fish Sauce	Read Ingredients	Yes					
Flax Seeds		Yes					

132

Flour								
	chestnut	No				*		
	amaranth	No				*		*
	arrowroot	Yes						
	barley	No				*		*
	buckwheat	Yes						
	coconut	No	*	*	*			
	corn	Yes						
	einkorn	No				*		
	emmer	No				*		
	green banana	Yes						
	lupin	No				*		*
	maize	Yes						
	millet	Yes						
	rice	Yes						
	rye	No				*		
	semolina (durum)	No				*		
	sorghum	Yes						
	spelt, organic	No				*		*
	spelt, organic, sieved	Yes						
	spelt, white	No				*		
	spelt, wholemeal	No				*		*
	teff	Yes						
	wheat	No				*		*
	yam	yes						
Flour Tortilla		No				*		
Fruit Juice		No						
Galangal		Yes						
Garlic		No				*		
Ginger Root		Yes						
Graham Crackers		No				*		

133

Item	Detail	Status					
Goji Berries	dried	No	*				
Grapefruit		No			*		
Grapes		Yes					
Green Onion						*	
	green part	Yes					
	white part	No			*		
Guava							
	ripe	Yes					
	canned in syrup	No	*		*		
Ham	check ingredients	Yes					
Hemp Seed		Yes					
High-Fructose Corn Syrup		No	*				
Honey		No	*				
horseradish		Yes					
Jackfruit		No	*		*		
jalapeño	pickled	Yes					
Jicama		Yes					
Kale		Yes					
Kiwi		Yes					
Kohlrabi		Yes					
Lamb		Yes					
Lays Potato Chips-original		Yes					
Leek Leaves							
	bulb	No			*		
	leaves	Caution		*			
Lemon		Yes					
Lemongrass		Yes					
Lentils		Caution					*
Lettuce	all types	Yes					
Lima Beans		No			*		*
Limes		Yes					
Longan		No		*	*		
Lotus Root							

	frozen	Yes						
	dried	No	*		*			
Lychee		No		*				
Mandarin Oranges		Yes						
Mangos		No	*					
Mangosteen								
	fresh	Yes						
	dried	No	*		*			
Maple Syrup		Yes						
Melon								
	Cantaloupe	Yes						
	Honeydew	No			*			
	Watermelon	No	*	*				*
Milk							*	
	A2	No					*	
	Almond	Yes						
	Buttermilk	No					*	
	Coconut-canned	Yes						
	Cow	No					*	
	Cream-cow	No					*	
	Cream-goat	No					*	
	Evaporated	No					*	
	Half & Half	Caution					*	
	Hemp	Yes						
	Kefir	No					*	
	Macadamia	Yes						*
	Oat	No						
	Quinoa	Yes						
	Rice	Yes						
	Soy (soy beans)	No						*
	Soy (soy protein)	Yes						
	Soya	No	*		*			*
	Sweetened Condensed	Yes						

Millet		Yes						
Mint		Yes						
Molasses		No	*		*		*	
Mushrooms								
	Oyster	Yes						
	Champignon, Button, Common - canned	Yes						
	Champignon, Button, Common	No		*	*			
	Enoki	No		*				
	Porcini-dried	No		*				
	Portobello - fresh	No		*				
	Shiitake	No		*				
	White back black, dried	Yes						
Mustard	read ingredients	Yes						
Mustard Greens		Yes						
Nectarines		No		*	*			
Noodles								
	laksa	No			*		*	
	brown rice vermicelli	Yes						
	kelp	Yes			*			
	rice	Yes						
	soba (made from wheat & buckwheat)	Yes						
	vermicelli	Yes						
	wheat	No	*		*			
Nutritional Yeast Flakes		Yes						
Nuts								
	Almonds	No					*	
	Brazil	Yes						
	Cashews	No			*		*	
	Chestnuts	Yes						
	Filberts (Hazelnuts)	Caution					*	
	Macadamia	Yes						
	Pecans	Yes						

136

Category	Item	Status					
	Pine Nuts	Yes					
	Pistachio	No			*		*
	Tigernuts	Yes					
	Walnuts	Yes					
Oats							
	flakes	Caution					*
	groats	Yes					
	coarse, organic	Yes					
	fine, organic	No			*		*
	gluten-free, organic, coarse	Yes					
	gluten-free, organic, fine	Caution			*		*
	quick	Caution			*		*
Okra		Yes					
Olives		Yes					
Onions							
	red	No			*		
	shallots	No			*		
	spring and scallion - bulb	No			*		
	spring and scallion - green tops only	Yes					
	white	No			*		*
	pickled, small	No	*				
Oranges		Yes					
Papaya					*		*
	fresh	Yes					
	dried	No			*		
Parsnip		Yes					
Passionfruit		Yes					
Pasta	check ingredients						
	chickpea	Yes					
	gluten free	Yes					
	gnocchi - wheat	No			*		

137

Category	Subtype	Yes/No						
	quinoa	Yes						
	spelt	No		*				
	wheat	No		*				
Peaches								
	clingstone	No	*					
	white	No	*	*				
	yellow	No	*					
	canned	No	*	*				
Peanut Butter	Read Ingredients	Yes						
Peanuts		Yes						
Pears		No	*	*				
Peas								
	green, canned	No					*	
	frozen	No		*			*	
	Sugar Snap	No	*					
	Snow	No	*	*			*	
Peppers, sweet, red								
peppers-hot								
Persimmons		No		*				
Pickles								
	Dill or Kosher							
	Sweet (including breading & butter)							
Pineapple								
	fresh	Yes						
	dried	No		*				
Pinto Beans		No						
Pistachios		No						
Plaintain		Yes						
Plums		No	*	*				
Polenta		Yes						
Pomegranates		No		*				
Poppy Seeds		Yes						

138

Pork		Yes					
Potatoes							
	sweet	Yes					
	unpeeled	Yes					
Potato Starch		Yes					
Prunes		No		*	*		
Pumpkin		Yes					
Pumpkin Seeds		Yes					
Quinoa		Yes					
Radicchio		Yes					
Radish		Yes					
Raisins		No		*	*		
	white (sultanas)	No	*		*		
Rambutan		No		*			
Raspberry		No			*		
Rhubarb		Yes					
Rhubarb		Yes					
Rice		Yes					
Rutabaga		Yes					
Rye Flour							
Salsify, black							
Sauerkraut		No		*			
Sausage							
Scallions							
Seafood		Yes	*				
Seaweed (Nori)	check ingredients	Yes					
Sesame Seeds		Yes					
Shallots							
Soda Pop	Not if there is HFCS, inverted sugar, or any bad sugars in it.						
Sour Cream		Yes					
Soy Beans						*	
Soy Sauce	I use gluten free	Yes			*		

Spelt		No			*		
Spices							
	All Spice	Yes					
	Asafoetida Powder (Hing) check ingredients, some use fillers	Yes					
	Basil-Dried	Yes					
	Basil-Fresh	Yes					
	Bay Leaves	Yes					
	Caraway Seeds	Caution				*	
	Chili Powder	Yes					
	Cilantro, fresh	Yes					
	Cinnamon, ground	Yes					
	Cloves	Yes					
	Coriander	Yes					
	Cumin	Yes					
	Curry	Yes	*				
	Dill	Yes					
	Fennel Seed	Yes					
	Five Spice	Yes					
	Ginger						
	Mustard Seed	Yes					
	Nutmeg	Yes					
	Oregano	Yes					
	Paprika	Yes					
	Parsley	Yes					
	Pepper, black	Yes					
	Poppy Seed	Yes					
	Rosemary	Yes					
	Saffron	Yes					
	Sage	Yes					
	Tarragon	Yes					
	Thyme	Yes					
	Turmeric	Yes					

140

Item	Variety/Notes	Safe					
Spinach		Yes					
Squash, winter							
	Butternut	No	*				
	Pattypan	Yes					
	Pumpkin	Yes					
	Spaghetti	Yes					
Starfruit		Yes					
Strawberries		Yes					
Sunflower seeds		Yes					
Sweet potatoes					*		
Swiss Chard	aka: chard, silverbeet	Yes					
Tamarind		Yes					
Tangerines (mandarin oranges)			*	*			
Tabioca Starch		Yes					
Taro		Yes					
Tea	weak	Yes		*			
Tempeh		Yes					
Tofu							
	firm, drained	Yes					
	plain	Yes					
	silken	No			*		*
Tomatoes							
	fresh	Yes					
	sundried	Caution	*				
Tomotillos							
	canned	Yes					
	fresh	No	*				
Turkey		Yes		*			
Turnip		Yes			*		
Vanilla		Yes					
Venison		Yes			*	*	
Vinegar						*	

141

Vinegar				*			
	Apple Cider	Yes					
	Balsamic	Caution	*				
	Malt	Yes					
	Rice Wine	Yes					
Wakame Flakes		Caution		*			
Wasabi		Yes					
Water Chestnut		Yes					
Watercress		Yes		*			
Watermelon		No	*		*		
Wheat		No	*		*		*
Wheat bread		No			*		*
Whipped Cream	real, read ingredient on processed	Yes					
Wine - Sweet					*		
Wonton Wrapper		Yes					
Worcestershire Sauce		Yes					
Yams		Yes					
Yogurt	Read Ingredients						
Zucchini		Caution			*		

Sources

Works Cited:

[1.] Barrett, Jacqueline S. & Gibson (sic?), Peter R. "Clinical Ramifications of Malabsorption of Fructose and Other Short Chain Carbohydrates" Practical Gastroenterology, August 2007. January 2008
http://www.healthsystem.virginia.edu/internet/digestive-health/nutrition/BarrettArticle.pdf

[2.] Corn Refiners Association "Nutritive Sweeteners from Corn" 2006, February 2008
http://www.corn.org/NSFC2006.pdf

[3.] Gotze, H. & Mahdi A., Comment in Monatsschr Kinderheilkd (German, translated), April 1993, February 2008
http://www.ncbi.nlm.nih.gov/pubmed/1470188?dopt=A

[4.] Kosmix Right Health, accessed February 2008
http://www.righthealth.com/Health/High__fructose__corn__syrup/-od-definition_wiki_High__fructose__corn__syrup-s

[5.] Ledochowski, Maximilian, Überall, Florian, Propst, Theresia, & Fuchs, Dietmar "Fructose Malabsorption Is Associated with Lower Plasma Folic Acid Concentrations

in Middle-Aged Subjects" Clinical Chemistry 1999, February   2008
http://www.clinchem.org/cgi/content/full/45/11/2013

6. Natoli, Sharon, "Fructose Malabsorption" Medical Observer, April 2006. February 2008
    <http://www.medicalobserver.com.au/displayarticle/index.asp?articleID=6260&templateID=108&sectionID=0&sectionName=

7. University of Virginia, Digestive Health Center "Low Fructose Diet" accessed February   2008
    <http://www.healthsystem.virginia.edu/internet/digestive-health/nutrition/low-fructose-diet.pdf
8. Nutritional Research Center.Org, "Health Tip #3",
http://nutritionresearchcenter.org/healthnews/health-tip-3-nix-high-fructose-corn-syrup/

9. Christian Antonioli, PhD candidate in psychiatry1, Michael A Reveley, professor of psychiatry1(june 2005)

10. Niedzielin K, Kordecki H, Birkenfeld B (2001). "A controlled, double-blind, randomized study on the efficacy of Lactobacillus **plantarum** 299V in patients with irritable bowel syndrome". Eur J Gastroenterol Hepatol 13 (10): 1143–7. doi:10.1097/00042737-200110000-00004. PMID 11711768. http://meta.wkhealth.com/pt/pt-core/template-

144

journal/lwwgateway/media/landingpage.htm?issn=0954-691X&volume=13&issue=10&spage=1143.

[11.] Boston University, HFI Laboratory
http://www.bu.edu/aldolase/HFI/treatment/sugar_table.htm

[12.] Prevention Magazine, March 2009, page 48

[13.] http://www.pulsus.com/cddw2007/abs/229
Fructose Malabsorption May Be Gender Dependent and
Fails to Show Compensation by Colonic Adaptation, A
Szilagyi, P Malolepszy, S Yesovitch, C Vinokuroff , U
Nathwani, A Cohen, X Xue
Division of Gastroenterology, Department of Medicine,
Department of Dietetics and Department of Emergency
Medicine, Sir Mortimer B Davis Jewish General
Hospital, McGill University, Montreal, Quebec

[14.] https://www.commonwealthfund.org/blog/2018/rising-obesity-
united-states-public-health-crisis, Apr 24, 2018

Other sources:

http://www.psychologyinfo.com/depression/

http://www.nimh.nih.gov/publicat/depression.cfm

http://www.dbsalliance.org/WPsearchable.pdf

http://www.mixednuts.net/depression-famous2.html

http://www.efmoody.com/longterm/depression.html

http://weblinks1.epnet.com GETTING DOWN TO DEPRESSION , By: Salmans, Sandra, Depression: Questions You Have...Answers You Need, 1997

FDA Consumer, May-June 2006

Harvard School of Public Health
http://www.hsph.harvard.edu/nutritionsource
and
www.thenutritionsource.org

Journal of Food Science
http://www3.interscience.wiley.com/journal/118832476/abstract

The World's Healthiest Foods website
http://whfoods.org/genpage.php?tname=nutrient&dbid=103#foodsources

http://www.raisin-hell.com/2008/11/fructans-inulin.html

http://www.sciencedaily.com/releases/2009/04/090420182151.htm

http://news.health.ufl.edu/news/story.aspx?ID=4992

Index

148

150

Made in the USA
Monee, IL
27 February 2021